Contents

Acknowledgements

Editor: Dr Annelies Wilder-Smith

Assistants: Christèle Wantz, Ruth Anderson

The following WHO personnel made contributions in their fields of expertise:

Dr Jorge Alvar
Dr Hoda Atta
Dr Bruce Aylward
Dr James Bartram
Dr Gautam Biswas
Dr Andrea Bosman
Dr Sylvie Briand
Dr Keith Carter
Dr Claire-Lise Chaignat
Dr Thomas Cherian
Dr Lester Chitsulo
Dr Eva-Maria Christophel
Dr Felicity Cutts
Dr Joelle Daviaud
Dr Neelam Dhingra-Kumar
Dr Micheline Diepart
Dr Philippe Duclos
Dr Mikhail Ejov
Dr Rainier Escalada
Dr Soce Fall
Dr Jan Fordham

Dr Pierre Formenty
Dr Ulrich Fruth
Dr Tracey Goodman
Dr Max Hardiman
Dr Frederick Hayden
Dr Joachim Hombach
Dr Janis K. Lazdins-Helds
Dr Lindsay Martinez
Dr Shanti Mendis
Dr François-Xavier Meslin
Dr Michael Nathan
Dr Kevin Palmer
Dr Margie Peden
Dr Aafje Rietveld
Dr Pascal Ringwald
Dr Cathy Roth
Dr Perez Simarro
Dr Rudolf Tangermann
Dr Krongthong Thimasarn
Dr David Wood

WHO gratefully acknowledges the collaboration of travel medicine experts and end-users of *International travel and health* who have provided advice and information for the 2007 edition:

Dr Paul Arguin, Chief, Domestic Response Unit, Malaria Branch, Division of Parasitic Diseases, Centers for Disease Control and Prevention, Atlanta, GA, USA

Dr Ron H. Behrens, Department of Travel Medicine, Hospital for Tropical Diseases, London, England

Dr Bjarne Bjorvatn, Professor, Centre for International Health, University of Bergen, Bergen, Norway

Dr Deborah J. Briggs, Professor, Department of Diagnostic Medicine/Pathobiology, College of Veterinary Medicine, Kansas State University, Manhattan, KS, USA

Dr Geneviève Brousse, Département des Maladies Infectieuses, Parasitaires, Tropicales et Santé Publique, Groupe Hospitalier Pitié-Salpêtrière, Paris, France

Dr Mads Buhl, Department of Infectious Diseases, Aarhus University Hospital, Aarhus, Denmark

Dr Martin Danis, Département des Maladies Infectieuses, Parasitaires, Tropicales et Santé Publique, Groupe Hospitalier Pitié-Salpêtrière, Paris, France

Mr Tom Frens, Managing Editor, Shoreland Inc., Milwaukee, WI, USA

Dr Anthony Gherardin, National Medical Adviser, Travel Doctor (TMVC) Group, Australia

Dr Peter Hackett, Altitude Research Center, University of Colorado Health Sciences Center, Aurora, CO, USA

Dr David Hill, Professor and Director, National Travel Health Network and Centre, London, England

Dr Shigeyuki Kano, Director, Department of Appropriate Technology, Development and Transfer, Research Institute, International Medical Center of Japan, Tokyo, Japan

Dr Phyllis E. Kozarsky, Professor of Medicine/Infectious Diseases, Director, Travel and Tropical Medicine, Emory University School of Medicine, Atlanta, GA, USA

Dr Louis Loutan, Associate Professor and Head, Travel and Migration Medicine Unit, Geneva University Hospitals, Geneva, Switzerland

Dr Anne McCarthy, Associate Professor, Tropical Medicine and International Health Clinic, Division of Infectious Diseases, Ottawa Hospital, Ottawa, Canada

Dr Ziad A. Memish, Director, Gulf Cooperation Council States Center for Infection Control, King Abdulaziz Medical City, Riyadh, Saudi Arabia

Dr Nebojša Nikoli, Medical Centre for Occupational Health Rijeka, Faculty of Maritime Studies, University of Rijeka, Rijeka, Croatia

Dr Hans D. Nothdurft, Professor and Head, University Travel Clinic, Department of Infectious Diseases and Tropical Medicine, University of Munich, Munich, Germany

Dr Walter Pasini, WHO Collaborating Centre for Tourist and Travel Medicine, Rimini, Italy

Dr Eskild Petersen, Head, Department of Mycobacteria and Parasitic Infections, Statens Serum Institute, Copenhagen, Denmark

Dr Christie Reed, Travelers' Health Team Lead, Centers for Disease Control and Prevention, Atlanta, GA, USA

Dr Lars Rombo, Clinic of Infectious Diseases, Eskilstuna, Sweden

Dr Patricia Schlagenhauf, Associate Professor, WHO Collaborating Centre for Travellers' Health, Institute of Social and Preventive Medicine, University of Zurich, Zurich, Switzerland

Dr Eli Schwartz, Associate Professor of Medicine at Sackler Faculty of Medicine, Tel-Aviv University; Head of the Center for Geographic Medicine and Tropical Diseases, Sheba Medical Center, Tel Hashomer, Israel

Dr Gerard Sonder, Landelijk Coördinatiecentrum Reizigersadvisering, Travel Clinic, Amsterdam, Netherlands

Dr Robert Steffen, Professor and Head, Division of Communicable Diseases, WHO Collaborating Centre for Travellers' Health, Institute of Social and Preventive Medicine, University of Zurich, Zurich, Switzerland

Dr Claude Thibeault, Medical Advisor, International Air Transport Association, Montreal, Canada

Dr Alfons Van Gompel, Head, Polyclinic-Travel Clinic, Institute of Tropical Medicine, Antwerp, Belgium

Dr Jane Zuckerman, Medical Director, Academic Centre for Travel Medicine and Vaccines and WHO Collaborating Centre for Travel Medicine, Royal Free and University College Medical School, London, England

Preface

International travel is undertaken by large, and ever increasing, numbers of people for professional, social, recreational and humanitarian purposes. More people travel greater distances and at greater speed than ever before, and this upward trend looks set to continue. Travellers are thus exposed to a variety of health risks in unfamiliar environments. Most such risks, however, can be minimized by suitable precautions taken before, during and after travel, and it is the purpose of this book to provide guidance on measures to prevent or reduce any adverse consequences for travellers' health.

The book is addressed primarily to medical and public health professionals who provide health advice to travellers, but it is also intended to provide guidance to travel agents and organizers, airlines and shipping companies. As far as possible, the information is presented in a form readily accessible to interested travellers and non-medical readers. For medical professionals, to whom other sources of additional material are available, essential information is given as concisely as possible.

The book is intended to give guidance on the full range of significant health issues associated with travel. The roles of the medical profession, the travel industry and travellers themselves in avoiding health problems are recognized. The recommendations address the health risks associated with different types of travel and travellers.

In this edition, emerging problems such as avian influenza and chikungunya have been added. Vaccine recommendations and schedules have been substantially revised and new vaccines are included. The chapter on malaria has been expanded to reflect current treatment options for malaria in travellers.

Air travel and its associated health risks receive emphasis, reflecting the enormous recent increase in travel by air, particularly long-haul flights. The passenger shipping industry (cruise ships and ferries) has expanded considerably in recent decades. In this edition, a section on travel by sea has been added to address the specific health issues involved. Business travel has increased dramatically, with frequent travellers now forming a substantial proportion of the total. Large numbers of travellers move far beyond the customary leisure and business centres, both for professional purposes and for pleasure, and there are now more elderly travellers, some of whom have pre-existing health problems. The risks and precautions specifically concerning infants and young children who travel also require special attention. An emerging subgroup of travellers — recent immigrants who return to their home countries for the purpose of visiting friends and relatives (VFR) — deserve a special section in this book because they are at a higher risk of certain health problems compared with traditional tourist and business travellers. A section on Hajj pilgrims has also been added.

Information is given on environmental factors that may have adverse effects on travellers' health and well-being. The main infectious diseases that pose potential health threats for travellers are described individually, with the corresponding preventive measures. The worldwide distribution of the major infectious diseases is shown in maps, and—where possible—extensive text has been replaced by lists and tables. A separate chapter is devoted to information on the vaccine-preventable diseases and the corresponding vaccines, as well as guidance on the selection of vaccines for individual travellers. Sources of additional information are included with each chapter.

The printed edition of this book is revised and published every year. An Internet version (www.who.int/ith) allows continuous updating and provides links to other information, such as news of current disease outbreaks of international importance.

CHAPTER I

Health risks and precautions: general considerations

The number of people travelling internationally is increasing every year. According to statistics of the World Tourism Organization, international tourist arrivals in the year 2005 exceeded 800 million. In 2005, the majority (402 million) of international tourist arrivals were for the purposes of leisure, recreation and holiday (50%). Business travel accounted for some 16% (125 million) and 26% (212 million) consisted of travel for other reasons such as visiting friends and relatives, religious purposes/pilgrimages and health treatment. For the remaining 8% of arrivals, the purpose of visit was not specified.

International travel can pose various risks to health, depending on the characteristics of both the traveller and the travel. Travellers may encounter sudden and significant changes in altitude, humidity, microbes and temperature, which can result in ill-health. In addition, serious health risks may arise in areas where accommodation is of poor quality, hygiene and sanitation are inadequate, medical services are not well developed and clean water is unavailable.

All people planning travel should know about the potential hazards of the countries they are travelling to and learn how to minimize their risk of acquiring these diseases. Forward planning, appropriate preventive measures and careful precautions can substantially reduce the risks of adverse health consequences. Although the medical profession and the travel industry can provide a great deal of help and advice, it is the traveller's responsibility to ask for information, to understand the risks involved, and to take the necessary precautions for the journey.

Travel-related risks

Key factors in determining the risks to which travellers may be exposed are:

— destination
— duration and season of travel
— purpose of travel
— standards of accommodation and food hygiene

— behaviour of the traveller
— underlying health of the traveller

Destinations where accommodation, hygiene and sanitation, medical care and water quality are of a high standard pose relatively few serious risks for the health of travellers, unless there is pre-existing illness. This also applies to business travellers and tourists visiting most major cities and tourist centres and staying in good-quality accommodation. In contrast, destinations where accommodation is of poor quality, hygiene and sanitation are inadequate, medical services do not exist, and clean water is unavailable may pose serious risks for the health of travellers. This applies, for example, to personnel from emergency relief and development agencies or tourists who venture into remote areas. In these settings, stringent precautions must be taken to avoid illness.

The epidemiology of infectious diseases in the destination country is of importance to travellers. Travellers and travel medicine practitioners should be aware of the occurrence of any disease outbreaks in their international destinations. New risks to international travellers may arise that are not detailed in this book. Unforeseen natural or manmade disasters may occur. Outbreaks of known or newly emerging infectious diseases are often unpredictable.

Emerging infectious diseases are commonly defined as:

— diseases that have newly appeared in a population;
— diseases that have existed in the past, but are rapidly increasing in incidence or geographical range.

The duration of the visit and the behaviour and lifestyle of the traveller are important in determining the likelihood of exposure to infectious agents and will influence decisions on the need for certain vaccinations or antimalarial medication. The duration of the visit may also determine whether the traveller may be subjected to marked changes in temperature and humidity during the visit, or to prolonged exposure to atmospheric pollution.

The purpose of the visit is critical in relation to the associated health risks. A business trip to a city, where the visit is spent in a hotel and/or conference centre of high standard, or a tourist trip to a well-organized resort involves fewer risks than a visit to a remote rural area, whether for work or pleasure. However, behaviour also plays an important role; for example, going outdoors in the evenings in a malaria-endemic area without taking precautions may result in the traveller becoming infected with malaria. Exposure to insects, rodents or other animals, infectious agents and contaminated food and water, combined with the absence of appropriate medical facilities, makes travel in many remote regions particularly hazardous.

Medical consultation before travel

Travellers intending to visit a destination in a developing country should consult a travel medicine clinic or medical practitioner before the journey. This consultation should take place at least 4–8 weeks before the journey, and preferably earlier if long-term travel or overseas work is envisaged. However, last-minute travellers can also benefit from a medical consultation, even as late as the day before travel. The consultation will determine the need for any vaccinations and/or antimalarial medication, as well as any other medical items that the traveller may require. A basic medical kit will be prescribed or provided, supplemented as appropriate to meet individual needs.

Dental and —for women— gynaecological check-ups are advisable before travel to developing countries or prolonged travel to remote areas. This is particularly important for people with chronic or recurrent dental or gynaecological/obstetric problems.

Assessment of health risks associated with travel

Medical advisers base their recommendations, including those for vaccinations and other medication, on an assessment of risk for the individual traveller, which takes into account the likelihood of catching a disease and how serious this might be for the traveller concerned. Key elements of this risk assessment are the destination, duration and purpose of the travel as well as the standards of accommodation and the health status of the traveller.

For each disease being considered, an assessment is also made of:

— availability of prophylaxis, possible side-effects and suitability for the traveller concerned;
— any associated public health risks (e.g. the risk of infecting others).

Collecting the information required to make a risk assessment involves detailed questioning of the traveller. A checklist or protocol is useful to ensure that all relevant information is obtained and recorded. The traveller should be provided with a personal record of the vaccinations given (patient-retained record) as vaccinations are often administered at different centres. A model checklist, reproducible for individual travellers, is provided.

Medical kit and toilet items

Sufficient medical supplies should be carried to meet all foreseeable needs for the duration of the trip.

3

A medical kit should be carried for all destinations where there may be significant health risks, particularly those in developing countries, and/or where the local availability of specific medications is not certain. This kit will include basic medicines to treat common ailments, first-aid articles, and any special medical items that may be needed by the individual traveller.

Certain categories of prescription medicine should be carried together with a medical attestation, signed by a physician, certifying that the traveller requires the medication for personal use. Some countries require not only a physician but also the national health administration to sign this certificate.

Toilet items should also be carried in sufficient quantity for the entire visit unless their availability at the travel destination is assured. These will include items for dental care, eye care including contact lenses, skin care and personal hygiene.

Contents of a basic medical kit

First-aid items:

- — adhesive tape
- — antiseptic wound cleanser
- — bandages
- — emollient eye drops
- — insect repellent
- — insect bite treatment
- — nasal decongestant
- — oral rehydration salts
- — scissors and safety pins
- — simple analgesic (e.g. paracetamol)
- — sterile dressing
- — clinical thermometer.

Additional items according to destination and individual needs:

- — antidiarrhoeal medication
- — antifungal powder
- — antimalarial medication
- — condoms
- — medication for any pre-existing medical condition
- — sedatives
- — sterile syringes and needles
- — water disinfectant

— other items to meet foreseeable needs, according to the destination and duration of the visit.

Travellers with pre-existing medical conditions and special needs

Special groups of travellers

Health risks associated with travel are greater for certain groups of travellers, including infants and young children, pregnant women, the elderly, the disabled, and those who have pre-existing health problems. Health risks may also differ depending on the purpose of travel, such as travel for the purpose of visiting friends and relatives (VFR) or for religious purposes/pilgrimages (Chapter 9), for relief work, or for business. For all of these travellers, medical advice and special precautions are necessary. They should be well informed about the available medical services at the travel destination.

Age

Infants and young children have special needs with regard to vaccinations and antimalarial precautions (see Chapters 6 and 7). They are particularly sensitive to ultraviolet radiation and become dehydrated more easily than adults in the event of inadequate fluid intake or loss of fluid due to diarrhoea. A child can be overcome by dehydration within a few hours. Air travel may cause discomfort to infants as a result of changes in cabin air pressure and is contraindicated for infants less than 48 hours old. Infants and young children are more sensitive to sudden changes in altitude. They are also more susceptible to infectious diseases.

Advanced age is not necessarily a contraindication for travel if the general health status is good. Elderly people should seek medical advice before planning long-distance travel.

Pregnancy

Travel is not generally contraindicated during pregnancy until close to the expected date of delivery, provided that the pregnancy is uncomplicated and the woman's health is good. Airlines impose some travel restrictions in late pregnancy and the neonatal period (see Chapter 2).

There are some restrictions on vaccination during pregnancy: specific information is provided in Chapter 6.

Pregnant women risk serious complications if they contract malaria. Travel to malaria-endemic areas should be avoided during pregnancy if at all possible. Specific recommendations for the use of antimalarial drugs during pregnancy are given in Chapter 7.

Medication of any type during pregnancy should be taken only in accordance with medical advice.

Travel to high altitudes (see also Chapter 3) or to remote areas is not advisable during pregnancy.

Disability

Physical disability is not usually a contraindication for travel if the general health status of the traveller is good. Airlines have regulations on the conditions for travel for disabled passengers who need to be accompanied (see Chapter 2). Information should be obtained from the airline in advance.

Pre-existing illness

People suffering from chronic illnesses should seek medical advice before planning a journey. Conditions that increase health risks during travel include:

— cardiovascular disorders
— chronic hepatitis
— chronic inflammatory bowel disease
— chronic renal disease requiring dialysis
— chronic respiratory diseases
— diabetes mellitus
— epilepsy
— immunosuppression due to medication or to HIV infection
— previous thromboembolic disease
— severe anaemia
— severe mental disorders
— any chronic condition requiring frequent medical intervention.

Any traveller with a chronic illness should carry all necessary medication for the entire duration of the journey. All medications, especially prescription medications, should be stored in carry-on luggage, in their original containers with clear labels. With heightened airline security, sharp objects will have to remain in checked luggage. Recently, airport security measures have introduced a restriction on liquids in carry-on luggage; it is therefore necessary to check with current airport security measures. A duplicate supply carried in the checked luggage is a safety precaution against loss or theft.

The traveller should carry the name and contact details of their physician on their person with other travel documents, together with information about the medical condition and treatment, and details of medication (generic drug names included) and prescribed doses. A physician's letter certifying the necessity for any drugs or other medical items (e.g. syringes) carried by the traveller that may be questioned by customs officials should also be carried.

Insurance for travellers

International travellers should be aware that medical care abroad is often available only at private medical facilities and may be costly. In places where good-quality medical care is not readily available, travellers may need to be repatriated in case of accident or illness. If death occurs abroad, repatriation of the body can be extremely expensive and may be difficult to arrange. Travellers should be advised (i) to seek information about possible reciprocal health-care agreements between the country of residence and the destination country, and (ii) to obtain special travellers' health insurance for destinations where health risks are significant and medical care is expensive or not readily available. This health insurance should include coverage for changes to the itinerary, emergency repatriation for health reasons, hospitalization, medical care in case of illness or accident and repatriation of the body in case of death.

Travel agents and tour operators usually provide information about travellers' health insurance. It should be noted that some countries now require proof of adequate health insurance as a condition for entry. Travellers should know the procedures to follow to obtain assistance and reimbursement. A copy of the insurance certificate and contact details should be carried with other travel documents in the hand luggage.

Role of travel industry professionals

Tour operators, travel agents, and airline and shipping companies each have an important responsibility to safeguard the health of travellers. It is in the interests of the travel industry that travellers have the fewest possible problems when travelling to, and visiting, foreign countries. Contact with travellers before the journey provides a unique opportunity to inform them of the situation in each of the countries they are visiting. The travel agent or tour operator should provide the following health-related guidance to travellers:

- Advise the traveller to consult a travel medicine clinic or medical practitioner as soon as possible after planning a trip to any destination where significant health risks may be foreseen, particularly those in developing countries, preferably 4–8 weeks before departure.

- Advise last-minute travellers that a visit should be made to a travel medicine clinic or medical practitioner, even up to the day before departure.
- Inform travellers if the destination presents any particular hazards to personal safety and security and suggest appropriate precautions.
- Encourage travellers to take out comprehensive travellers' health insurance and provide information on available policies.
- Inform travellers of the procedures for obtaining assistance and reimbursement, particularly if the insurance policy is arranged by the travel agent or company.
- Provide information on:
  - mandatory vaccination requirements for yellow fever;
  - the need for malaria precautions at the travel destination;
  - the existence of other important health hazards at the travel destination;
  - the presence or absence of good-quality medical facilities at the travel destination.

Responsibility of the traveller

Travellers can obtain a great deal of information and advice from medical and travel industry professionals to help prevent health problems while abroad. However, travellers must accept that they are responsible for their health and well-being while travelling and on their return. The following are the main responsibilities to be accepted by the traveller:

- the decision to travel
- recognition and acceptance of any risks involved
- seeking health advice in good time, preferably 4–8 weeks before travel
- compliance with recommended vaccinations and other prescribed medication and health measures
- careful planning before departure
- carrying a medical kit and understanding its use
- obtaining adequate insurance cover
- health precautions before, during and after the journey
- responsibility for obtaining a physician's letter pertaining to any prescription medicines, syringes, etc. being carried
- responsibility for the health and well-being of accompanying children

— precautions to avoid transmitting any infectious disease to others during and after travel
— careful reporting of any illness on return, including information about all recent travel
— respect for the host country and its population.

A model checklist for use by travellers, indicating steps to be taken before the journey, is provided at the end of the chapter.

Medical examination after travel

Travellers should be advised to have a medical examination on their return if they:

— suffer from a chronic disease, such as cardiovascular disease, diabetes mellitus, chronic respiratory disease;
— experience illness in the weeks following their return home, particularly if fever, persistent diarrhoea, vomiting, jaundice, urinary disorders, skin disease or genital infection occurs;
— consider that they have been exposed to a serious infectious disease while travelling;
— have spent more than 3 months in a developing country.

Travellers should provide medical personnel with information on recent travel, including destination, and purpose and duration of visit. Frequent travellers should give details of all journeys that have taken place in the preceding weeks and months.

Note. Fever after returning from a malaria-endemic area is a medical emergency and travellers should seek medical attention immediately.

Further reading

Keystone JS et al., eds. *Travel medicine*, 1st ed. London, Elsevier, 2004.

Overview International Tourism 2005, UN World Tourism Organization: http://www.unwto.org/facts/menu.html

Steffen R, Dupont HL, Wilder-Smith A, eds. *Manual of travel medicine and health*, 2nd ed. London, BC Decker, 2007.

Zuckerman JN, ed. *Principles and practice of travel medicine*. Chichester, Wiley, 2001.

Checklist for the traveller

Obtain information on local conditions

Depending on destination

- Risks related to the area (urban or rural)
- Type of accommodation (hotel, camping)
- Length of stay
- Altitude
- Security problems (e.g. conflict)
- Availability of medical facilities

Prevention

Vaccination. Contact the nearest travel medicine centre or a physician as early as possible, preferably 4–8 weeks before departure.

Malaria. Request information on malaria risk, prevention of mosquito bites, possible need for appropriate preventive medication and emergency reserves, and plan for bednet and insect repellent.

Food hygiene. Eat only thoroughly cooked food and drink only well-sealed bottled or packaged cold drinks. Boil drinking-water if safety is doubtful. If boiling is not possible, a certified well-maintained filter and/or disinfectant agent can be used.

Specific local diseases. Consult the appropriate sections of this volume.

Accidents related to:

- Traffic (obtain a card showing blood group before departure)
- Animals (beware of snakes and rabid dogs)
- Allergies (use a medical alert bracelet)
- Sun (pack sunglasses and sunscreen)

Get the following check-ups

- Medical—obtain prescriptions for medication according to length of stay, and obtain advice from your physician on assembling a suitable medical kit
- Dental
- Ophthalmological—pack spare spectacles
- Other according to specific conditions (e.g. pregnancy, diabetes)

Subscribe to a medical insurance with appropriate cover abroad, i.e. accident, sickness, medical repatriation.

Pre-departure medical questionnaire

Surname: First name:

Date of birth: Country of origin:

Purpose of travel: ☐ Private   ☐ Professional

Special activities: ☐ Accommodation: e.g. camping, bivouac

                            ☐ Sports: e.g. diving, hunting, high-altitude trekking

Date of departure and length of stay:

Places to be visited

Country	Town	Rural area		Dates	
		Yes	No	From	to
		Yes	No	From	to
		Yes	No	From	to
		Yes	No	From	to
		Yes	No	From	to

Medical history:

Vaccination record:

Current state of health:

Chronic illnesses:

Recent or current medical treatment:

History of jaundice or hepatitis:

Allergies (e.g. eggs, antibiotics, sulfonamides):

For women: ☐ Current pregnancy

                 ☐ Pregnancy likely within 3 months

                 ☐ Currently breastfeeding

History of anxiety or depression:

                 ☐ If yes, treatment prescribed (specify)

Neurological disorders (e.g. epilepsy, multiple sclerosis, etc.):

Cardiovascular disorders (e.g. thrombosis, use of pacemaker):

CHAPTER 2

Mode of travel: health considerations

The mode of travel is an integral part of the travel experience. According to the World Tourism Organization (UNWTO), of the 800 million international tourist arrivals in 2005, air transport represented 45% of arrivals and transport over water accounted for 7%. This chapter deals with travel by air and by sea. Travel by air and by sea expose passengers to a number of factors that may have an impact on health.

Travel by air

This section was prepared in collaboration with the International Civil Aviation Organization and the International Air Transport Association. To facilitate use by a wide readership, technical terms have been used sparingly. Medical professionals needing more detailed information are referred to the website of the Aerospace Medical Association: www.asma.org.

The volume of air traffic has risen steeply in recent years and the number of long-distance flights has greatly increased. With modern long-range aircraft, the need for "stop-overs" has been reduced so the duration of flights has also increased. The passenger capacity of long-distance aircraft is also growing, and larger numbers of people travel aboard a single aircraft. "Frequent flyers" now make up a substantial proportion of the travelling public. According to the International Civil Aviation Organization, the annual number of air passengers reached 2 billion in 2005, and passenger traffic is projected to grow by about 6% a year over the period 2006–2008.

Air travel, in particular over long distances, exposes passengers to a number of factors that may have an effect on their health and well-being. Passengers with pre-existing health problems are more likely to be affected and should consult their doctor or a travel medicine clinic in good time before travelling. Those receiving medical care and intending to travel by air in the near future should tell their medical adviser. Health risks associated with air travel can be minimized if the traveller plans carefully and takes some simple precautions before, during and after the flight. An explanation of the various factors that may affect the health and well-being of air travellers follows.

Cabin air pressure

Although aircraft cabins are pressurized, cabin air pressure at cruising altitude is lower than air pressure at sea level. At typical cruising altitudes in the range 11 000–12 200 metres (36 000–40 000 feet) air pressure in the cabin is equivalent to the outside air pressure at 1800–2400 metres (6000–8000 feet) above sea level. As a consequence, less oxygen is taken up by the blood (hypoxia) and gases within the body expand. The effects of reduced cabin air pressure are usually well tolerated by healthy passengers.

Oxygen and hypoxia

Cabin air contains ample oxygen for healthy passengers and crew. However, because cabin air pressure is relatively low, the amount of oxygen carried in the blood is reduced compared with sea level. Passengers with certain medical conditions, particularly heart and lung disease and blood disorders such as anaemia, may not tolerate this reduced oxygen level (hypoxia) very well. Such passengers are usually able to travel safely if arrangements are made with the airline for the provision of an additional oxygen supply during flight.

Gas expansion

As the aircraft climbs, the decreasing cabin air pressure causes gases to expand. Similarly, as the aircraft descends, the increasing pressure in the cabin causes gases to contract. These changes may have effects where gas is trapped in the body.

Gas expansion during the climb causes air to escape from the middle ear and the sinuses, usually without causing problems. This airflow can sometimes be perceived as a "popping" sensation in the ears. As the aircraft descends, air must flow back into the middle ear and sinuses in order to equalize pressure differences. If this does not happen, the ears or sinuses may feel as if they are blocked and, if the pressure is not relieved, pain can result. Swallowing, chewing or yawning ("clearing the ears") will usually relieve any discomfort. If the problem persists, a short forceful expiration against a pinched nose and closed mouth (Valsalva manoeuvre) will usually help. For infants, feeding or giving a pacifier (dummy) to stimulate swallowing may reduce the symptoms.

Individuals with ear, nose and sinus infections should avoid flying because pain and injury may result from the inability to equalize pressure differences. If travel cannot be avoided, the use of decongestant nasal drops shortly before the flight and again before descent may be helpful.

As the aircraft climbs, expansion of gas in the abdomen can cause discomfort, although this is usually mild.

Some forms of surgery, other medical treatments or diagnostic tests may introduce air or other gas into a body cavity. Examples include abdominal surgery or eye treatment for a detached retina. Passengers who have recently undergone such a procedure should ask a travel medicine physician or their treating physician how long they should wait before undertaking air travel.

Cabin humidity and dehydration

The humidity in aircraft cabins is low, usually less than 20% (humidity in the home is normally over 30%). Low humidity may cause skin dryness and discomfort of the eyes, mouth, nose and exposed skin but presents no risk to health. Using a skin moisturizing lotion, saline nasal spray to moisturize the nasal passages, and spectacles rather than contact lenses can relieve or prevent discomfort. The low humidity does not cause internal dehydration and there is no need to drink extra water.

Ozone

Ozone is a form of oxygen (with three, rather than two, atoms to the molecule) that occurs in the upper atmosphere and may enter the aircraft cabin together with the fresh air supply. In older aircraft, it was found that the levels of ozone in cabin air could sometimes lead to irritation of the lungs, eyes and nasal tissues. Ozone is broken down by heat and most ozone is removed by the compressors (in the aircraft engines) that provide pressurized air for the cabin. In addition, most modern long-haul jet aircraft are fitted with equipment (catalytic converters) that breaks down any remaining ozone.

Cosmic radiation

Cosmic radiation is made up of radiation that comes from the sun and from outer space. The earth's atmosphere and magnetic field are natural shields and cosmic radiation levels are therefore lower at lower altitudes. Cosmic radiation is more intense over polar regions than over the equator because of the shape of the earth's magnetic field and the "flattening" of the atmosphere over the poles.

The population is continually exposed to natural background radiation from soil, rock and building materials as well as from cosmic radiation that reaches the earth's surface. Although cosmic radiation levels are higher at aircraft cruising altitudes than at sea level, research has not shown any significant health effects for either passengers or crew.

Motion sickness

Except in the case of severe turbulence, travellers by air rarely suffer from motion (travel) sickness. Those who do suffer should request a seat in the mid-section of the cabin where movements are less pronounced, and keep the motion sickness bag, provided at each seat, readily accessible. They should also consult their doctor or travel medicine physician about medication that can be taken before flight to help prevent problems, and should avoid drinking alcohol during the flight and for the 24 hours beforehand.

Immobility, circulatory problems and deep vein thrombosis (DVT)

Contraction of muscles is an important factor in helping to keep blood flowing through the veins, particularly in the legs. Prolonged immobility, especially when seated, can lead to pooling of blood in the legs, which in turn may cause swelling, stiffness and discomfort.

It is known that immobility is one of the factors that may lead to the development of a blood clot in a deep vein, so-called "deep vein thrombosis" or DVT. Research has shown that DVT can occur as a result of prolonged immobility, for instance during long-distance travel, whether by car, bus, train or air. The World Health Organization has set up a major research study (WRIGHT) to confirm the association between air travel and deep vein thrombosis and to find out whether there are any factors that might lead to the risk of DVT being higher for air travel than for other causes of immobility.

In most cases of DVT, the clots are small and do not cause any symptoms. The body is able to gradually break down the clots and there are no long-term effects. Larger clots may cause symptoms such as swelling of the leg, tenderness, soreness and pain. Occasionally a piece of the clot may break off and travel with the bloodstream to become lodged in the lungs. This is known as pulmonary embolism and may cause chest pain, shortness of breath and, in severe cases, sudden death. This can occur many hours or even days after the formation of the clot.

The risk of developing DVT when travelling is increased in the presence of other risk factors, including:

— previous DVT or pulmonary embolism;

- history of DVT or pulmonary embolism in a close family member;
- use of estrogen therapy – oral contraceptives ("the Pill") or hormone replacement therapy (HRT);
- pregnancy;
- recent surgery or trauma, particularly to the abdomen, pelvic region or legs;
- cancer;
- obesity;
- some inherited blood-clotting abnormalities.

It is advisable for people with one or more of these risk factors to seek specific medical advice from their doctor or a travel medicine clinic in good time before embarking on a flight of three or more hours.

DVT occurs more commonly in older people. Some researchers have suggested that there may be a risk from smoking and from varicose veins.

Precautions

The benefits of most precautionary measures in passengers at particular risk for DVT are unproven and some might even result in harm. However, some general advice for such passengers is given here.

Moving around the cabin during long flights will help to reduce any period of prolonged immobility, although this may not always be possible. Moreover, any potential health benefits must be balanced against the risk of injury if the aircraft were to experience sudden turbulence. A sensible compromise may be to make regular trips to the bathroom, e.g. every 2–3 hours. Many airlines also provide helpful advice on exercises that can be carried out in the seat during flight. It is thought that exercise of the calf muscles can stimulate the circulation, alleviate discomfort, fatigue and stiffness, and may reduce the risk of developing DVT. Hand luggage should not be placed where it restricts movement of the legs and feet, and clothing should be loose and comfortable.

In view of the clear risk of significant side-effects and absence of clear evidence of benefit, passengers are advised not to use aspirin specifically for the prevention of travel-related DVT.

Those travellers who are at most risk of developing DVT may be prescribed specific treatments and should consult their doctor for further advice.

Diving

Divers should avoid flying soon after diving because of the risk that the reduced cabin pressure may lead to decompression sickness (the bends). It is recommended that they do not fly until at least 12 hours after the last dive and this period should be extended to 24 hours after multiple dives or after diving that requires decompression stops during ascent to the surface. Passengers undertaking recreational diving before flying should seek specialist advice from diving schools.

Jet lag

Jet lag is the term used for the symptoms caused by the disruption of the body's "internal clock" and the approximate 24-hour (circadian) rhythms it controls. Disruption occurs when crossing multiple time zones, i.e. when flying east to west or west to east. Jet lag may lead to indigestion and disturbance of bowel function, general malaise, daytime sleepiness, difficulty in sleeping at night, and reduced physical and mental performance. Its effects are often combined with tiredness caused by the journey itself. Jet lag symptoms gradually wear off as the body adapts to the new time zone.

Jet lag cannot be prevented but there are ways of reducing its effects (see below). Travellers who take medication according to a strict timetable (e.g. insulin, oral contraceptives) should seek medical advice from their doctor or a travel medicine clinic before their journey.

General measures to reduce the effects of jet lag

- Be as well rested as possible before departure, and rest during the flight. Short naps can be helpful.

- Eat light meals and limit consumption of alcohol. Alcohol increases urine output, with the result that sleep may be disturbed by the need to urinate. While it can accelerate the onset of sleep, alcohol impairs the quality of sleep, making sleep less restorative. The after-effects of excessive consumption of alcohol ("hangover") can exacerbate the effects of jet lag and travel fatigue. Alcohol should therefore be consumed in moderation, if at all, before and during flight. Caffeine should be limited to normal amounts and avoided within a few hours of an expected period of sleep.

- Try to create the right conditions when preparing for sleep. When taking a nap during the day, eyeshades and earplugs may help. Regular exercise during the day may help to promote sleep, but avoid strenuous exercise immediately before sleep.

- At the destination, try to get as much sleep in every 24 hours as normal. A minimum block of 4 hours' sleep during the local night – known as "anchor sleep" – is thought to be necessary to allow the body's internal clock to adapt to the new time zone. If possible, make up the total sleep time by taking naps during the day in response to feelings of sleepiness.

- The cycle of light and dark is one of the most important factors in setting the body's internal clock. Exposure to daylight at the destination will usually help adaptation.

- Short-acting sleeping pills may be helpful. They should be used only in accordance with medical advice and should not normally be taken during the flight, as they may increase immobility and therefore the risk of developing DVT.

- Melatonin is available in some countries and can be used to help resynchronize the body's internal clock. It is normally sold as a food supplement and therefore is not subject to the same strict control as medications (for example, it has not been approved for use as a medication in the United States, but can be sold as a food supplement). The timing and effective dosage of melatonin have not been fully evaluated and its side-effects, particularly in long-term use, are unknown. Moreover, manufacturing methods are not standardized: the dose in each tablet can be very variable and some harmful compounds may be present. For these reasons, melatonin cannot be recommended.

- It is not always appropriate to adjust to local time for short trips of up to 2–3 days . If in doubt, seek specialist travel medicine advice.

- Individuals react in different ways to time zone changes. Frequent flyers should learn how their own bodies respond and adopt habits accordingly. Advice from a travel medicine clinic may help in formulating an effective coping strategy.

Psychological aspects

Travel by air is not a natural activity for humans and many people experience some degree of psychological difficulty when flying. The main problems encountered are stress and fear of flying. These may occur together or separately at different times before and during the period of travel.

Stress

All forms of travel generate stress. Flying can be particularly stressful because it often involves a long journey to the airport, curtailed sleep and the need to walk long distances in the terminal building. Most passengers find their own ways of coping, but passengers who find air travel particularly stressful should seek medical advice in good time. Good planning (passports, tickets, medication, etc.) and allowing plenty of time to get to the airport help to relieve stress.

Flight phobia (fear of flying)

Fear of flying may range from feeling slightly anxious to being unable to travel by air at all. It can lead to problems at work and leisure.

Travellers who want to travel by air but are unable to do so because of their fear of flying should seek medical advice before the journey. Medication may be useful in some cases, but the use of alcohol to "steady the nerves" is not helpful and may be dangerous if combined with some medicines. For a longer-term solution, travellers should seek specialized treatment to reduce the psychological difficulties associated with air travel. There are many courses available that aim to reduce, or cure, the fear of flying. These typically include advice on how to cope with the symptoms of fear, information about how an aircraft flies, how controls are operated during a flight, and, in most cases, a short flight.

Air rage

In recent years, air rage has been recognized as a form of disruptive behaviour associated with air travel. It appears to be linked to high levels of general stress but not specifically to flight phobia. It is frequently preceded by excessive consumption of alcohol.

Travellers with medical conditions or special needs

Airlines have the right to refuse to carry passengers with conditions that may worsen, or have serious consequences, during the flight. They may require medical clearance from their medical department/adviser if there is an indication that a passenger could be suffering from any disease or physical or mental condition that:

— may be considered a potential hazard to the safety of the aircraft;
— adversely affects the welfare and comfort of the other passengers and/or crew members;
— requires medical attention and/or special equipment during the flight;
— may be aggravated by the flight.

If cabin crew suspect before departure that a passenger may be ill, the aircraft's captain will be informed and a decision taken as to whether the passenger is fit to travel, needs medical attention, or presents a danger to other passengers and crew or to the safety of the aircraft.

Although this chapter provides some general guidelines on conditions that may require medical clearance in advance, airline policies do vary and requirements should always be checked at the time of, or before, booking the flight. A good place to find information is often the airline's own web site.

Infants

A fit and healthy baby can travel by air 48 hours after birth, but it is preferable to wait until the age of 7 days when possible. Until their organs have developed properly and stabilized, premature babies should always undergo a medical clearance before travelling by air. Changes in cabin air pressure may upset infants; this can be helped by feeding or giving a pacifier (dummy) to stimulate swallowing.

Pregnant women

Pregnant women can normally travel safely by air, but most airlines restrict travel in late pregnancy. Typical guidelines for a woman with an uncomplicated pregnancy are:

— after the 28th week of pregnancy, a letter from a doctor or midwife should be carried, confirming the expected date of delivery and that the pregnancy is normal;
— for single pregnancies, flying is permitted up to the end of the 36th week;
— for multiple pregnancies, flying is permitted up to the end of the 32nd week.

Each case of complicated pregnancy requires medical clearance.

Pre-existing illness

Most people with medical conditions are able to travel safely by air, provided that necessary precautions, such as the need for additional oxygen supply, are considered in advance.

Those who have underlying health problems such as cancer, heart or lung disease, anaemia and diabetes, who are on any form of regular medication or treatment, who have recently had surgery or have been in hospital, or who are concerned about their fitness to travel for any other reason should consult their doctor or a travel medicine clinic before deciding to travel by air.

Medication that may be required during the journey, or soon after arrival, should be carried in the hand luggage. It is also advisable to carry a copy of the prescription in case the medication is lost, additional supplies are needed or security checks require proof of purpose.

Frequent travellers with medical conditions

A frequent traveller who has a permanent and stable underlying health problem may obtain a frequent traveller's medical card from the medical or reservation department of many airlines. This card is accepted, under specified conditions, as proof of medical clearance and for identification of the holder's medical condition.

Dental/oral surgery

Recent dental work such as fillings is not usually a contraindication to flying. However, unfinished root canal treatment and abscessed tooth are reasons for caution, and it is recommended that each individual seek advice with regard to travel plans from the surgeon or dental practitioner most familiar with their case.

Security issues

Security checks can cause concerns for travellers who have been fitted with metal devices such as artificial joints, pacemakers or internal automatic defibrillators. Some pacemakers may be affected by modern security screening equipment and any traveller with a pacemaker should carry a letter from their doctor. Travellers who need to carry other medical equipment in their hand luggage, particularly sharp items such as hypodermic needles, should also carry a letter from their doctor.

Smokers

Almost all airlines now ban smoking on board. Some smokers may find this stressful, particularly during long flights, and should discuss this with a doctor before travelling. Nicotine replacement patches or chewing gum containing nicotine may be helpful during the flight and the use of other medication or techniques may also be considered.

Travellers with disabilities

A physical disability is not usually a contraindication for travel. A passenger who is unable to look after his or her own needs during the flight (including use of the toilet and transfer from wheelchair to seat and vice versa) will need to be accompanied by an escort able to provide all necessary assistance. The cabin crew are generally not permitted to provide such assistance and a traveller who requires it but does not have a suitable escort may not be permitted to travel. Travellers confined to wheelchairs should be advised against deliberately restricting fluid intake before or during travel as a means of avoiding use of toilets during flights as this may be detrimental to overall health.

Airlines have regulations on conditions of travel for passengers with disabilities. Disabled passengers should contact airlines in advance of travel for guidance; the airlines' own web sites often give useful information.

Communicable diseases

Research has shown that there is very little risk of any communicable disease being transmitted on board the aircraft.

The quality of aircraft cabin air is carefully controlled. Ventilation rates provide a total change of air 20–30 times per hour. Most modern aircraft have recirculation systems, which recycle up to 50% of cabin air. The recirculated air is usually passed through HEPA (high-efficiency particulate air) filters, of the type used in hospital operating theatres and intensive care units, which trap particles, bacteria, fungi and viruses.

Transmission of infection may occur between passengers who are seated in the same area of an aircraft, usually as a result of the infected person coughing or sneezing or by touch (direct contact or contact with the same parts of the aircraft cabin and furnishings that other passengers touch). This is no different from any other situation in which people are close to each other, such as on a train or bus or at a theatre. Highly contagious conditions, such as influenza, are more likely to be spread to other passengers in situations when the aircraft ventilation system is not operating. An auxiliary power unit is normally used to provide ventilation when the aircraft is on the ground, before the main engines are started, but occasionally this is not operated for environmental (noise) or technical reasons. In such cases, when associated with a prolonged delay, passengers may be temporarily disembarked.

Transmission of tuberculosis (TB) on board commercial aircraft during long-distance flights was reported during the 1980s, but no case of active TB disease resulting from exposure on board has been identified subsequently. Nevertheless, increasing air travel and the emergence of multidrug-resistant and extensively drug-resistant TB require continuing vigilance to avoid the spread of infection during air travel.

During the outbreak of severe acute respiratory syndrome (SARS) in 2003, the risk of transmission of SARS in aircraft was very low.

To minimize the risk of passing on infections, passengers who are unwell, particularly if they have a fever, should delay their journey until they have recovered. Passengers with a known active communicable disease should not travel by air. Airlines may deny boarding to passengers who appear to be infected with a communicable disease.

Aircraft disinsection

Many countries require disinsection of aircraft (to kill insects) arriving from countries where diseases that are spread by insects, such as malaria and yellow fever, occur. There have been a number of cases of malaria affecting individuals who live or work in the vicinity of airports in countries where malaria is not present, thought to be due to the escape of malaria-carrying mosquitoes transported on aircraft. Some countries, e.g. Australia and New Zealand, routinely carry out disinsection to prevent the inadvertent introduction of species that may harm their agriculture.

Disinsection is a public health measure that is mandated by the International Health Regulations (see Annex 2). It involves treatment of the interior of the aircraft with insecticides specified by WHO. The different procedures currently in use are as follows:

— treatment of the interior of the aircraft using a quick-acting insecticide spray immediately before take-off, with the passengers on board;
— treatment of the interior of the aircraft on the ground before passengers come on board, using a residual-insecticide aerosol, plus additional in-flight treatment with a quick-acting spray shortly before landing;
— regular application of a residual insecticide to all internal surfaces of the aircraft, except those in food preparation areas.

Travellers are sometimes concerned about their exposure to insecticide sprays during air travel, and some have reported feeling unwell after spraying of aircraft for disinsection. However, WHO has found no evidence that the specified insecticide sprays are harmful to human health when used as prescribed.

Medical assistance on board

Airlines are required to provide minimum levels of medical equipment on aircraft and to train all cabin crew in first aid. The equipment carried varies, with many airlines carrying more than the minimum level of equipment required by the regulations. Equipment carried on a typical international flight would include:

— one or more first-aid kits, to be used by the crew;
— a medical kit, normally to be used by a doctor or other qualified person, to treat in-flight medical emergencies;

An automated external defibrillator (AED), to be used by the crew in case of cardiac arrest, is also carried by several airlines.

Cabin crew are trained in the use of first-aid equipment and in carrying out first-aid and resuscitation procedures. They are usually also trained to recognize a range of medical conditions that may cause emergencies on board and to act appropriately to manage these.

In addition, many airlines have facilities to enable crew to contact a medical expert at a ground-based response centre for advice on how to manage in-flight medical emergencies.

Contraindications to air travel

Travel by air is normally contraindicated in the following cases:

- Infants less than 48 hours old.

- Women after the 36th week of pregnancy (after 32nd week for multiple pregnancies).

- Those suffering from:
  — angina pectoris or chest pain at rest;
  — any active communicable disease;
  — decompression sickness after diving;
  — increased intracranial pressure due to haemorrhage, trauma or infection;
  — infections of the sinuses or of the ear and nose, particularly if the Eustachian tube is blocked;
  — recent myocardial infarction and stroke (time period depending on severity of illness and duration of travel);
  — recent surgery or injury where trapped air or gas may be present, especially abdominal trauma and gastrointestinal surgery, craniofacial and ocular injuries, brain operations, and eye operations involving penetration of the eyeball;
  — severe chronic respiratory disease, breathlessness at rest, or unresolved pneumothorax;

— sickle-cell disease;
— psychotic illness, except when fully controlled.

The above list is not comprehensive, and fitness for travel should be decided on a case-by-case basis.

Further reading

International Civil Aviation Organization: http://icao.int

Medical guidelines for airline travel, 2nd ed. Alexandria, VA, Aerospace Medical Association, Medical Guidelines Task Force, 2003; available at http://www.asma.org/pdf/publications/medguid.pdf.

Mendis S, Yach D, Alwan Al. Air travel and venous thromboembolism. *Bulletin of the World Health Organization,* 2002, 80(5):403–406.

Report of WHO Research into Global Hazards of Travel (WRIGHT) Project 2006. Geneva, World Health Organization (in preparation)

Summary of SARS and air travel. Geneva, World Health Organization, 23 May 2003; available at http://www.who.int/csr/sars/travel/airtravel/en/

The impact of flying on passenger health: a guide for healthcare professionals, London, British Medical Association, Board of Science and Education, 2004; available at http://www.bma.org.uk/ap.nsf/AttachmentsByTitle/PDFFlying/$FILE/Impactofflying.pdf.

Tourism highlights: 2006 edition. Madrid, World Tourism Organization, 2006; available at http://www.unwto.org/facts/menu.html

Tuberculosis and air travel: guidelines for prevention and control, 2nd ed. Geneva, World Health Organization, 2006 (WHO/HTM/TB/2006.363).

Travel by sea

This section was prepared in collaboration with the International Society of Travel Medicine.

The passenger shipping industry (cruise ships and ferries) has expanded considerably in recent decades. In 2005, 11.5 million passengers worldwide travelled on cruise ships. Cruise itineraries include all continents including areas that are not easily accessible by other means of travel. The average duration of a cruise is about 7 days, but cruise voyages can last from several hours to several months (e.g. round-the-world cruises).

The revised International Health Regulations (2005) address health requirements for ship operations and construction. There are global standards regarding ship and port sanitation and disease surveillance, as well as response to infectious diseases. Guidance is given on provision of safe water and food, on vector and rodent control, and on waste disposal. According to Article 8 of the International Labour Organization Convention (No. 164) "Concerning Health Protection and Medical Care for Seafarers" (1987), vessels carrying more than 100 crew members on an international voyage of three days or longer must provide a physician for care of the crew. These regulations do not apply to passenger vessels and ferries sailing for less than three days, even though the number of crew and passengers may exceed 1000. The contents of the ship's medical chest must be in accordance with the international agreements for ocean-going trade vessels but there are no special requirements for additional drugs for passenger ships.

Industry-wide, the average traveller on a cruise line is 45–50 years of age. Cruises of longer duration often attract older travellers, a group likely to have more chronic medical problems, such as heart and lung disease, which may worsen during travel. Extended periods away from the home port, especially days at sea, make it essential for passengers to stock up with sufficient medical supplies. Prescription medicines should be carried in the original packages or containers, together with a letter from a medical practitioner attesting to the traveller's need for those medicines. Cruise ship travellers who have chronic diseases, who require more comprehensive facilities than are available on the ship or who may require particular medical treatment should consult their health-care providers. Knowledge of the types and quality of medical facilities along the itinerary is important to determine whether travellers or crew members can be sent ashore for additional care or need to be evacuated by air back to the home port. It is important to view a ship's medical facility as an infirmary and not a hospital. Although most of the medical conditions that arise aboard ship can be treated as they would at an ambulatory care centre at home, more severe problems may require the patient to be treated in a fully staffed and equipped land-based hospital after stabilization on the ship.

The rapid movement of cruise ships from one port to another, with the likelihood of wide variations in sanitation standards and infectious disease exposure risks, often results in the introduction of communicable diseases by embarking passengers and crew members. In the relatively closed and crowded environment of a ship, disease may well spread to other passengers and crew members; diseases may also be disseminated to the home communities of disembarking passengers and crew members. A literature review by WHO identified more than 100 disease outbreaks associated with ships since 1970. This is probably an underestimate because many outbreaks are not reported and some may go undetected. Such outbreaks are of concern because of their potentially serious health consequences and high costs to the industry. Outbreaks of measles, rubella, varicella, meningococcal meningitis, hepatitis A, legionellosis, and respiratory and gastrointestinal illnesses among ship travellers have been reported. In recent years, influenza and norovirus outbreaks have been public health challenges for the cruise industry.

Communicable diseases

Gastrointestinal disease

Most of the detected gastrointestinal disease outbreaks associated with cruise ships have been linked to food or water consumed on board ship. Factors that have contributed to outbreaks include contaminated bunkered water, inadequate disinfection of water, potable water contaminated by sewage on ship, poor design and construction of storage tanks for potable water, deficiencies in food handling, preparation and cooking, and use of seawater in the galley. Norovirus is the most common pathogen implicated in outbreaks. Symptoms often start with sudden onset of vomiting and/or diarrhoea. There may be fever, abdominal cramps and malaise. The virus can spread in food or water or from person to person; it is highly infectious and in an outbreak on a cruise ship in 1998, more than 80% of the 841 passengers were affected. To prevent or reduce outbreaks of gastroenteritis caused by norovirus, some cruise companies ask that those who present with gastrointestinal symptoms at on-board medical centres are put in isolation until at least 24 hours after their last symptoms, and some ships also isolate asymptomatic contacts for 24 hours.

Influenza and other respiratory tract infections

Respiratory tract infections are frequent among cruise-ship travellers. Travelling in large groups may pose a risk of exposure to influenza viruses in regions of the world where influenza is not in seasonal circulation, particularly if the group contains travellers from areas of the world where influenza viruses are in seasonal circulation. Crew members who serve passengers may become reservoirs for influenza infection and may transmit disease to passengers on subsequent cruises.

Legionellosis

Legionellosis (Legionnaires' disease) is a potentially fatal form of pneumonia, first recognized in 1976. The disease is normally contracted by inhaling *Legionella* bacteria deep into the lungs. *Legionella* species can be found in tiny droplets of water (aerosols) or in droplet nuclei (the particles left after water has evaporated). The WHO literature review showed that more than 50 incidents of legionellosis, involving over 200 cases, have been associated with ships during the past three decades. For example, an outbreak of legionellosis occurred on a single cruise ship in 1994, resulting in 50 passengers becoming affected on nine separate cruises, with one death. The disease was linked to a whirlpool spa on the ship.

Prevention and control depend on proper disinfection, filtration and storage of source water; avoidance of dead ends in pipes and regular cleaning and disinfection of spas are required to reduce the risk of legionellosis on ships.

Noncommunicable diseases

Because of temperature and weather variations, changes in diet and physical activities, and generally increased levels of stress compared with life at home, the cruise ship traveller – particularly the elderly traveller – may experience worsening of existing chronic health conditions. Cardiovascular events are the most common cause of mortality on cruise ships. Motion sickness can occur, especially on smaller vessels.

Precautions

The risk of communicable and noncommunicable diseases among cruise ship passengers and crew members is difficult to quantify because of the broad spectrum of cruise ship experiences, the variety of destinations and the limited available data. In general, prospective cruise ship travellers should:

— ensure that they are up to date with all routinely recommended age- and medical condition-specific immunizations;
— consider influenza vaccination regardless of season, particularly if they belong to groups for whom annual vaccination against influenza is routinely recommended (see Chapter 6);
— follow the prevention and immunization recommendations that apply to each country on the itinerary;
— carry out frequent hand-washing, either with soap and water or using an alcohol-based hand sanitizer;
— consult a physician or travel health specialist who may provide prevention guidelines and immunizations according to the health status of the cruise ship traveller, the duration of travel, countries to be visited and likely activities ashore;
— consult a physician or travel medicine specialist about medication against motion sickness, particularly if they are prone to motion sickness;
— carry all prescription medicines in the original packet or container, together with a physician's letter;

— consult their health-care provider before embarking on a cruise if they have any health conditions that might increase the potential for illness on a cruise ship;

— consult a physician to determine the individual risk of serious complications of influenza and the need to provide a prescription for anti-influenza medication, for treatment or prophylaxis.

Further reading

American College of Emergency Physicians: http://www.acep.org/webportal/membercenter/sections/cruise/

International Council of Cruise Lines: http://www.iccl.org/policies/medical.cfm

International Maritime Health Association: http://www.imha.net/

Miller JM et al. Cruise ships: high-risk passengers and the global spread of new influenza viruses. *Clinical Infectious Diseases*, 2000, 31:433–438

Sanitation on ships. Compendium of outbreaks of foodborne and waterborne disease and Legionnaires' disease associated with ships: 1970–2000. Geneva, World Health Organization, 2001 (WHO/SDE/WSH/01.4).

Sherman CR. Motion sickness: review of causes and preventive strategies. *Journal of Travel Medicine*, 2002, 9:251–256

Ship sanitation and health: http://www.who.int/mediacentre/factsheets/fs269/en/

Smith A. Cruise ship medicine. In: Dawood R, ed. *Travellers' health*. Oxford, Oxford University Press, 2002:277–289.

CHAPTER 3

Environmental health risks

Travellers often experience abrupt and dramatic changes in environmental conditions, which may have detrimental effects on health and well-being. Travel may involve major changes in altitude, temperature and humidity, and exposure to microbes, animals and insects. The negative impact of sudden changes in the environment can be minimized by taking simple precautions.

Altitude

Barometric pressure falls with increasing altitude, diminishing the partial pressure of oxygen and causing hypoxia. The partial pressure of oxygen at 2500 m, the altitude of Vail, Colorado, for example, is 26% lower than at sea level; in La Paz, Bolivia (4000 m), it is 41% lower. This places a substantial stress on the body, which requires at least a few days to acclimatize; the extent of acclimatization may be limited by certain medical conditions, especially lung disease. An increase in alveolar oxygen through increased ventilation is the key to acclimatization; this process starts at 1500 m. Despite successful acclimatization, aerobic exercise performance remains impaired and travellers may still experience problems with sleep.

High-altitude illness (HAI) results when hypoxic stress outstrips acclimatization. HAI can occur at any altitude above 2100 m, but is particularly common above 2750 m. In Colorado ski resorts, incidence of HAI varies from 15% to 40%, depending on sleeping altitude. Susceptibility is primarily genetic, but fast rates of ascent and higher sleeping altitudes are important precipitating factors. Age, sex and physical fitness have little influence.

The spectrum of HAI includes common acute mountain sickness (AMS), occasional high-altitude pulmonary oedema and, rarely, high altitude cerebral oedema. The latter two conditions, although uncommon, are potentially fatal. AMS may occur after 1–12 hours at high altitude. Headache is followed by anorexia, nausea, insomnia, fatigue and lassitude. Symptoms usually resolve spontaneously in 24–48 hours and are ameliorated by oxygen or analgesics and antiemetics. Acetazolamide 5 mg/kg per day in divided doses is an effective chemoprophylaxis for all HAI; it is started one day before travel to altitude and continued for the first two days at altitude.

Only a few conditions are contraindications for travel to altitude; they include unstable angina, pulmonary hypertension, severe chronic obstructive pulmonary disease (COPD) and sickle-cell disease. Patients with stable coronary disease, hypertension, diabetes, asthma or mild COPD, and pregnant women generally tolerate altitude well but may require monitoring of their condition. Portable and stationary oxygen supplies are readily available in most high-altitude resorts and – by removing hypoxic stress – remove any potential danger from altitude exposure.

Precautions for travellers unaccustomed to high altitudes

- Avoid one-day travel to sleeping altitudes over 2750 m if possible. Break the journey for at least one night at 2000–2500 m to help prevent AMS.

- Avoid overexertion and alcohol for the first 24 hours at altitude, drink extra water.

- If direct travel to sleeping altitude over 2750 m is unavoidable, consider prophylaxis with acetazolamide.

- Acetazolamide is also effective if started early in the course of AMS.

- Travellers planning to climb or trek at high altitude will require a period of gradual acclimatization.

- Travellers with pre-existing cardiovascular or pulmonary disease should seek medical advice before travelling to high altitudes.

- Travellers with the following symptoms should seek medical attention when, at altitude:
  - symptoms of AMS that are severe or last longer than 2 days
  - progressive shortness of breath with cough and fatigue
  - ataxia or altered mental status.

Heat and humidity

Sudden changes in temperature and humidity may have adverse effects on health. Exposure to high temperature and humidity results in loss of water and electrolytes (salts) and may lead to heat exhaustion and heat stroke. In hot dry conditions, dehydration is particularly likely to develop unless care is taken to maintain adequate fluid intake. The addition of a little table salt to food or drink (unless this is contraindicated for the individual) can help to prevent heat exhaustion, particularly during the period of adaptation.

Consumption of salt-containing food and drink helps to replenish the electrolytes in case of heat exhaustion and after excessive sweating. Older travellers should take particular care to consume extra fluids in hot conditions, as the thirst reflex diminishes with age. Care should be taken to ensure that infants and young children drink enough liquid to avoid dehydration.

Irritation of the skin may be experienced in hot conditions (prickly heat). Fungal skin infections such as tinea pedis (athlete's foot) are often aggravated by heat and humidity. A daily shower, wearing loose cotton clothing and applying talcum powder to sensitive skin areas help to reduce the development or spread of these infections.

Exposure to hot, dry, dusty air may lead to irritation and infection of the eyes and respiratory tract.

Ultraviolet radiation from the sun

The ultraviolet (UV) radiation from the sun includes UVA (wavelength 315–400 nm) and UVB (280–315 nm) radiation, both of which are damaging to human skin and eyes. The intensity of UV radiation is indicated by the Global Solar UV Index, which is a measure of skin-damaging radiation. The Index describes the level of solar UV radiation at the Earth's surface and is often reported as the maximum 10–30-minute average for the day. The values of the Index range from zero upwards—the higher the Index value, the greater the potential for damage to the skin and eyes, and the less time it takes for harm to occur. The Index values are grouped into exposure categories, with values greater than 10 being "extreme". In general, the closer to the equator the higher the Index. UVB radiation is particularly intense in summer and in the 4-hour period around solar noon. UV radiation may penetrate clear water to a depth of 1 metre or more.

The adverse effects of ultraviolet radiation from the sun are the following:

- Exposure to UV radiation, particularly UVB, can produce severe debilitating sunburn and sunstroke, particularly in light-skinned people.

- Exposure of the eyes may result in acute keratitis ("snow blindness"), and long-term damage leads to the development of cataracts.

- Long-term adverse effects on the skin include:
  - the development of skin cancers (carcinomas and malignant melanoma), mainly due to UVB radiation;
  - accelerated ageing of the skin, mainly due to UVA radiation, which penetrates more deeply into the skin.

- Adverse reactions of the skin result from interaction with a wide range of medicinal drugs that may cause photosensitization and result in phototoxic or photoallergic dermatitis. A variety of different types of therapeutic drugs as well as oral contraceptives, some prophylactic antimalarial drugs and certain antimicrobials may cause adverse dermatological reactions on exposure to sunlight. Phototoxic contact reactions are caused by topical application of products, including perfumes, containing oil of bergamot or other citrus oils.

- Exposure may suppress the immune system, increase the risk of infectious disease, and limit the efficacy of vaccinations.

Precautions

- Avoid exposure to the sun in the middle of the day, when the UV intensity is greatest.

- Wear clothing that covers arms and legs (summer clothing is UV-protective and generally more effective than even good-quality sunscreen).

- Wear UV-protective sunglasses of wrap-around design and a wide-brimmed sun hat.

- Apply a broad-spectrum sunscreen of sun protection factor (SPF) 15+ liberally on areas of the body not protected by clothing and reapply frequently.

- Take particular care to ensure that children are well protected.

- Take precautions against excessive exposure on or in water.

- Check that medication being taken will not affect sensitivity to UV radiation.

- If adverse skin reactions have occurred previously, avoid any exposure to the sun and avoid any products that have previously caused the adverse reactions.

Foodborne and waterborne health risks

Many important infectious diseases (such as brucellosis, cholera, cryptosporidiosis, giardiasis, hepatitis A and E, legionellosis, leptospirosis, listeriosis, schistosomiasis and typhoid fever) are transmitted by contaminated food and water. Information on these and other specific infectious diseases of interest for travellers is provided in Chapter 5.

For travellers, the main health problem associated with contaminated food and water is "travellers' diarrhoea", which can be caused by a wide range of infectious agents. Travellers' diarrhoea is the most common health problem encountered by travellers and may affect up to 80% of travellers to high-risk destinations. Even a brief episode of severe diarrhoea may spoil a holiday or ruin a business trip. Diarrhoea may be accompanied by nausea, vomiting and fever. Travellers' diarrhoea is primarily the result of consumption of contaminated food, drink or drinking-water. Contamination in such cases is due to the presence of disease-producing microorganisms. A wide range of different bacteria and viruses, and some parasitic and fungal infections may cause travellers' diarrhoea.

Illness is also caused by certain biological toxins found in seafood. The main diseases in this group are caused by poisoning from:

— paralytic shellfish
— neurotoxic shellfish
— amnesic shellfish
— ciguatera toxin
— scombroid fish
— puffer fish.

The toxins involved in these poisonings come from microorganisms consumed by or otherwise contaminating the fish.

Poisonous chemicals may also contaminate food and drink. However, the ill-effects are generally the result of long-term exposure and do not represent a significant health risk for travellers. Sporadic misuse of chemicals also occurs, such as the use of textile dyes in foodstuffs, which may give an unusually bright colour to the contaminated food.

The safety of food, drink and drinking-water depends mainly on the standards of hygiene applied locally in their preparation and handling. In countries with low standards of hygiene and sanitation and poor infrastructure for controlling the safety of food, drink and drinking-water, there is a high risk of contracting travellers' diarrhoea. In such countries, travellers should take precautions with **all** food and drink, including that served in good-quality hotels and restaurants, to minimize any risk of contracting a foodborne or waterborne infection. While the risks are greater in poor countries, locations with poor hygiene may be present in any country. Another potential source of waterborne infection is contaminated recreational water (see next section),

It is particularly important that people in more vulnerable groups, i.e. infants and children, the elderly, pregnant women and people with impaired immune systems, take stringent precautions to avoid contaminated food and drink and unsafe recreational waters.

Precautions for avoiding unsafe food and drink

- Avoid cooked food that has been kept at room temperature for several hours.
- Eat only food that has been cooked thoroughly and is still hot.

Intestinal parasites: risks for travellers

Travellers, particularly those visiting tropical and subtropical countries, may be exposed to a number of intestinal parasitic helminth (worm) infections. The risk of acquiring intestinal parasites is associated with low standards of hygiene and sanitation, which permit contamination of soil, sand and foodstuffs with human or canine faeces. In general, the clinical effects are likely to become apparent some time after return from travel and the link with the travel destination may not be apparent, which in turn may delay the diagnosis or lead to misdiagnosis. The following are the main intestinal parasitic helminths to which travellers may be exposed.

■ **Hookworms**. Human and canine hookworms, particularly *Necator* and *Ancylostoma* species, may be a risk for travellers, notably in places where beaches are polluted by human or canine faeces. Humans become infected by larval forms of the parasite which penetrate the skin. *A. caninum* produces a characteristic skin lesion, cutaneous larval migrans, which is readily treated by anthelminthics such as albendazole.

■ **Tapeworms**. The tapeworm *Taenia saginata* is acquired by consumption of raw or undercooked beef from cattle that harbour the larval form of the parasite. *T. solium* is similarly acquired from raw or undercooked pork. These tapeworm infections result from access of cattle and pigs to human faeces, from which they ingest tapeworm eggs. *T. solium* infection in humans may also result from ingestion of *T. solium* eggs in food contaminated by faeces; this is particularly dangerous, since the larval forms of the parasite cause cysticercosis, which may produce serious disease. The tapeworm *Echinococcus granulosum* causes cystic hydatid disease due to infection by the larval form of the parasite; the adult tapeworms infect dogs, which excrete eggs in the faeces. Human infection is acquired by ingestion of eggs following close contact with infected dogs or consumption of food or water contaminated by their faeces.

■ **Roundworms**. The intestinal roundworm (nematode) parasites *Ascaris* and *Trichuris* are transmitted in soil. Soil containing eggs of these parasites may contaminate foods such as fruit and vegetables, leading to infection if the food is consumed without thorough washing; infection may also be transmitted by the hands following handling of soil-contaminated foods, for instance in street markets.

- Avoid uncooked food, apart from fruit and vegetables that can be peeled or shelled, and avoid fruits with damaged skins.
- Avoid dishes containing raw or undercooked eggs.
- Avoid food bought from street vendors.
- Avoid ice cream from unreliable sources, including street vendors.
- In countries where poisonous biotoxins may be present in fish and shellfish, obtain advice locally.
- Boil unpasteurized (raw) milk before consumption.
- Boil drinking-water if its safety is doubtful; if boiling is not possible, a certified, well-maintained filter and/or a disinfectant agent can be used.
- Avoid ice unless it has been made from safe water.
- Avoid brushing the teeth with unsafe water.
- Bottled or packaged cold drinks are usually safe provided that they are sealed; hot beverages are usually safe.

Treating water of questionable quality

- Bringing water to a rolling boil is the most effective way to kill all disease-causing pathogens. Let the hot water cool down on its own without adding ice (as one cannot be sure if the ice itself is safe).
- If it is not possible to boil water, chemical disinfection of clear, non-turbid water is effective for killing bacteria and viruses and some protozoa (but not, for example, *Cryptosporidium*). Chlorine and iodine are the chemicals most commonly used for disinfection.
- A product that combines chlorine disinfection with coagulation/flocculation (i.e., chemical precipitation) should be used, when available, as these products remove significant numbers of protozoa, in addition to killing bacteria and viruses.
- If turbid water (i.e. not clear, or with suspended solid matter) is to be disinfected with chemicals, it should be cleared beforehand, for example by letting the impurities settle or by filtering.
- Portable point-of-use (POU) devices tested and rated to remove protozoa and some bacteria are also available. Ceramic, membrane and carbon-block filters are the most common types. Selecting the most appropriate filter pore size is crucial; a size of 1 μm or less for the filter media pore is recommended to ensure removal of *Cryptosporidium* in clear water.

- Unless water is boiled, a combination of methods (e.g. filtration followed by chemical disinfection or boiling) is recommended, since most POU filtration devices do not remove nor kill viruses. Reverse osmosis (very fine pore filtration that holds back dissolved salts in the water) and ultrafiltration (fine pore filtration that passes dissolved salts but holds back viruses and other microbes) devices can theoretically remove all pathogens.

- Often, after chemical treatment, a carbon filter is used to improve taste and, in the case of iodine treatment, to remove excess iodine.

Treatment of diarrhoea

Most diarrhoeal episodes are self-limiting, with recovery in a few days. It is important, especially for children, to avoid becoming dehydrated.

As soon as diarrhoea starts, more fluids should be taken, such as safe water (bottled, boiled or chlorinated). If diarrhoea continues for more than one day, oral rehydration salt (ORS) solution should be taken and normal food consumption should continue.

Amounts of ORS solution to drink

Children under 2 years	$^1/_4$–$^1/_2$ cup (50–100 ml) after each loose stool up to approximately 0.5 litre a day.
Children 2–9 years	$^1/_2$–1 cup (100–200 ml) after each loose stool up to approximately 1 litre a day.
Patients of 10 years or older	As much as wanted, up to approximately 2 litres a day.

If ORS solution is not available, a substitute containing 6 level teaspoons of sugar plus 1 level teaspoon of salt in 1 litre of safe drinking-water can be used, in the same amounts as for ORS. (A level teaspoon contains a volume of 5 ml.)

Medical help should be sought if diarrhoea lasts for more than 3 days and/or there are very frequent watery bowel movements, blood in the stools, repeated vomiting or fever.

When medical help is not available, first-line antibiotics such as fluoroquinolones (e.g. ciprofloxacin or levofloxacin) can be used as empirical therapy. However, increasing resistance to fluoroquinolones, especially among *Campylobacter* isolates, may lower their efficacy in some parts of the world, particularly in Asia. In such cases, azithromycin can be taken as an alternative treatment. Azithromycin is also the first-line antibiotic therapy for children and pregnant women. When immediate relief of diarrhoea is needed in travellers, antidiarrhoeal drugs such as loperamide may be additionally used, but such antimotility drugs are contraindicated in children.

Prophylactic use of antibiotics is not recommended. Prophylactic use of antidiarrhoeal medicines is always contraindicated.

Breastfeeding should not be interrupted.

In case of any other symptoms, medical advice should be sought rapidly.

Recreational waters

The use of coastal waters and freshwater lakes and rivers for recreational purposes has a beneficial effect on health through exercise, and rest and relaxation. However, various hazards to health may also be associated with recreational waters. The main risks are the following:

- Drowning and injury (see Chapter 4).
- Physiological:
  - chilling, leading to coma and death;
  - thermal shock, leading to cramps and cardiac arrest;
  - acute exposure to heat and ultraviolet radiation in sunlight: heat exhaustion, sunburn, sunstroke;
  - cumulative exposure to sun (skin cancers, cataract).
- Infection:
  - ingestion or inhalation of, or contact with, pathogenic bacteria, fungi, parasites and viruses;
  - bites by mosquitoes and other insect vectors of infectious diseases.
- Poisoning and toxicoses:
  - ingestion or inhalation of, or contact with, chemically contaminated water, including oil slicks;
  - stings or bites of venomous animals;
  - ingestion or inhalation of, or contact with, blooms of toxigenic plankton.

Exposure to cold: immersion hypothermia

Cold, rather than simple drowning, is the main cause of death at sea. When the body temperature falls (hypothermia), there is confusion followed by loss of consciousness, so that the head goes under water leading to drowning. With a life jacket capable of keeping the head out of water, drowning is avoided, but death due directly to hypothermic cardiac arrest will soon follow. However, wearing warm clothing as well as a life jacket can greatly prolong survival in cold water. Children, particularly boys, have less fat than adults and chill very rapidly in cool or cold water.

Swimming is difficult in very cold water (around 0 °C), and even good swimmers often drown suddenly if they attempt to swim even short distances in water at these temperatures without a life jacket. Life jackets or some other form of flotation aid should always be worn in small craft, particularly by children and young men, when the water is cold.

Alcohol, even in small amounts, can cause hypoglycaemia if consumed without food and after exercise. It causes confusion and disorientation and also, in cold surroundings, a rapid fall in body temperature. Unless sufficient food is eaten at the same time, small amounts of alcohol can be exceedingly dangerous on long-distance swims, as well as after rowing or other strenuous and prolonged water-sports exercise.

Those engaging in winter activities on water, such as skating and fishing, should be aware that whole-body immersion must be avoided. Accidental immersion in water at or close to freezing temperatures is dangerous because the median lethal immersion time (time to death) is less than 30 minutes for children and most adults.

Immediate treatment is much more important than any later action in reviving victims of immersion hypothermia. A hot bath (the temperature no higher than the immersed hand will tolerate) is the most effective method of achieving this. In case of drowning, cardiac arrest and cessation of breathing should be treated by tipping water out of the stomach and giving immediate external cardiac massage and artificial ventilation. Cardiac massage should not be applied unless the heart has stopped. People who have inhaled water should always be sent to hospital to check for pulmonary complications.

Infection

In coastal waters, infection may result from ingestion or inhalation of, or contact with, pathogenic microorganisms, which may be naturally present, carried by people or animals using the water, or present as a result of faecal contamination.

The most common consequences among travellers are diarrhoeal disease, acute febrile respiratory disease and ear infections.

In fresh waters, leptospirosis may be spread by the urine of infected rodents, causing human infection through contact with broken skin or mucous membranes. In areas endemic for schistosomiasis, infection may be acquired by penetration of the skin by larvae during swimming or wading. (See also Chapter 5.)

In swimming pools and spas, infection may occur if treatment and disinfection of the water are inadequate. Diarrhoea, gastroenteritis and throat infections may result from contact with contaminated water. Appropriate use of chlorine and other disinfectants controls most viruses and bacteria in water. However, the parasites *Giardia* and *Cryptosporidium*, which are shed in large numbers by infected individuals, are highly resistant to routine disinfection procedures. They are inactivated by ozone or eliminated by filtration.

Contamination of spas and whirlpools may lead to infection by *Legionella* and *Pseudomonas aeruginosa*. Otitis externa and infections of the urinary tract, respiratory tract, wounds and cornea have also been linked to spas.

Direct person-to-person contact or physical contact with contaminated surfaces in the vicinity of pools and spas may spread the viruses that cause molluscum contagiosum and cutaneous papillomas (warts); fungal infections of the hair, fingernails and skin, notably tinea pedis (athlete's foot), are spread in a similar manner.

Precautions

- Adopt safe behaviour in all recreational waters (see Chapter 4).
- Avoid consumption of alcohol before any activities in or near recreational waters.
- Provide constant supervision of children in the vicinity of recreational waters.
- Avoid temperature extremes in spas, saunas, etc; this is particularly important for users with pre-existing medical conditions, pregnant women and young children.
- Avoid excessive exposure to sunlight.
- Avoid contact with contaminated waters.
- Avoid swallowing any contaminated water.

- Obtain advice locally about the presence of potentially dangerous aquatic animals.
- Wear shoes when walking on shores, riverbanks and muddy terrain.

Animals and insects

Mammals

Animals tend to avoid contact with humans and most do not attack unless provoked. Some large carnivores, however, are aggressive and may attack. Animals suffering from rabies often become aggressive and may attack without provocation. Wild animals may become aggressive if there is territorial intrusion, particularly when the young are being protected. Animal bites may cause serious injury and may also result in transmission of disease.

Rabies is the most important infectious health hazard from animal bites. In many developing countries, rabies is transmitted mainly by dogs, but many other species of mammals can be infected by the rabies virus. After any animal bite, the wound should be thoroughly cleansed with disinfectant or with soap or detergent and water, and medical or veterinary advice should be sought about the possibility of rabies in the area. Where a significant risk of rabies exists, the patient should be treated with post-exposure rabies vaccination and immunoglobulin (see Chapter 5). A booster dose of tetanus toxoid is also recommended following an animal bite.

Travellers who may be at increased risk of exposure to rabies may be advised to have pre-exposure vaccination before departure (see Chapter 6). Pre-exposure rabies vaccination does not eliminate the need for treatment after the bite of a rabid animal, but it reduces the number of vaccine doses required in the post-exposure regimen.

Precautions

- Avoid direct contact with domestic animals in areas where rabies occurs, and with all wild and captive animals.
- Avoid behaviour that may startle, frighten or threaten an animal.
- Ensure that children do not approach, touch or otherwise provoke any animal.
- Treat any animal bite immediately by washing with disinfectant or soap and seek medical advice.

INTERNATIONAL TRAVEL AND HEALTH 2007

- If a significant risk of exposure to rabies is foreseen, seek medical advice before travelling.

Travellers with accompanying animals should be aware that dogs (and, for some countries, cats) must be vaccinated against rabies in order to be allowed to cross international borders. A number of rabies-free countries have additional requirements. Before taking an animal abroad, the traveller should ascertain the regulatory requirements of the countries of destination and transit.

Snakes, scorpions and spiders

Travellers to tropical, subtropical and desert areas should be aware of the possible presence of venomous snakes, scorpions and spiders. Local advice should be sought about risks in the areas to be visited. Most venomous species are particularly active at night.

Venom from snake and spider bites and from scorpion stings has various effects in addition to tissue damage in the vicinity of the bite. Neurotoxins are present in the venom of both terrestrial and aquatic snakes, and also often in the venom of scorpions and spiders. Neurotoxins cause weakness and paralysis and other symptoms. Venom contacting the eyes causes severe damage and may result in blindness. Most snake venoms affect blood coagulation, which may result in haemorrhage and reduced blood pressure. Toxins in the hair of spiders such as tarantulas may cause intense irritation on contact with the skin.

Poisoning by a venomous snake, scorpion or spider is a medical emergency requiring immediate attention. The patient should be moved to the nearest medical facility as quickly as possible. First-aid measures call for immobilizing the entire affected limb with splints and firm, but not tight, bandaging to limit the spread of toxin in the body and the amount of local tissue damage. However, bandaging is not recommended if local swelling and tissue damage are present in the vicinity of the bite. Other traditional first-aid methods (incisions and suction, tourniquets and compression) are harmful and should not be used.

The decision to use antivenom should be taken only by qualified medical personnel, and it should be administered in a medical facility. Antivenom should be given only if its stated range of specificity includes the species responsible for the bite.

Precautions
- Obtain local advice about the possible presence of venomous snakes, scorpions and spiders in the area.

- Avoid walking barefoot or in open sandals in terrain where venomous snakes, scorpions or spiders may be present; wear boots or closed shoes and long trousers.
- Avoid placing hands or feet where snakes, spiders or scorpions may be hiding.
- Be particularly careful outdoors at night.
- Examine clothing and shoes before use for hidden snakes, scorpions or spiders.

Aquatic animals

Swimmers and divers may be bitten by certain aquatic animals, including conger and moray eels, stingrays, weever fish, scorpionfish, stonefish, piranhas, seals and sharks. They may be stung by venomous cnidaria—jellyfish, fire corals, sea anemones—and other invertebrate aquatic species including octopus. Severe and often fatal injury results from attack by crocodiles, which inhabit rivers and estuaries in many tropical countries, including the tropical north of Australia. Injuries from dangerous aquatic organisms occur as a result of:

- passing close to a venomous organism while bathing or wading;
- treading on a stingray, weever fish or sea urchin;
- handling venomous organisms during sea-shore exploration;
- invading the territory of large animals when swimming or at the water's edge;
- swimming in waters used as hunting grounds by large predators;
- interfering with, or provoking, dangerous aquatic organisms.

Precautions

- Obtain local advice on the possible presence of dangerous aquatic animals in the area.
- Adopt behaviour that will avoid provoking attack by predatory animals.
- Wear shoes when walking on the shore and at the water's edge.
- Avoid contact with jellyfish in water and dead jellyfish on the beach.
- Avoid walking, wading or swimming in crocodile-infested waters at all times of year.
- Seek medical advice after a sting or bite by a poisonous animal.

Treatment

In the case of envenomings by aquatic animals, treatment will depend on whether there is a wound or puncture or a localized skin reaction (e.g. rash). Punctures caused by spiny fish require immersion in hot water, extraction of the spines, careful cleaning of the wound and antibiotic therapy (and antivenom in the case of stonefish). If punctures were caused by an octopus or sea urchin the treatment is basically the same but without exposure to heat. In the case of rashes or linear lesions, contact with cnidaria should be suspected; the treatment is based on the use of 5% acetic acid, local decontamination and corticosteroids (antivenom for the box jellyfish *Chironex fleckeri*), with adequate follow-up for eventual sequelae.

Insects and other vectors of disease

Vectors play an essential role in the transmission of many infectious diseases. Many vectors are bloodsucking insects, which ingest the disease-producing microorganism during a blood meal from an infected host (human or animal) and later inject it into a new host at the time of another blood meal. Mosquitoes are important insect vectors of disease, and some diseases are transmitted by bloodsucking flies. In addition, ticks and certain aquatic snails are involved in the life cycle and transmission of disease. The principal vectors and the main diseases they transmit are shown in Table 3.1 at the end of this chapter. Information about the diseases and specific preventive measures are provided in Chapters 5, 6 and 7.

Water plays a key role in the life cycle of most vectors. Thus, the transmission of many vector-borne diseases is seasonal as there is a relationship between rainfall and the existence of breeding sites. Temperature is also a critical factor, limiting the distribution of vectors by altitude and latitude.

Travellers are usually at lower risk of exposure to vector-borne diseases in urban centres, especially if they sleep in air-conditioned rooms. They may, however, be exposed to the vectors of dengue which are frequent in urban centres in tropical countries and which bite mostly during the day. Travellers to rural areas or to areas with low standards of hygiene and sanitation are usually at higher risk of exposure to disease vectors and personal protection is therefore essential. Evening/night-time activities outdoors may increase exposure to malaria vectors.

Protection against vectors

Travellers may protect themselves from mosquitoes and other vectors by the means outlined in the following paragraphs.

Insect repellents are substances applied to exposed skin or to clothing to prevent human/vector contact. The active ingredient in a repellent repels but does not kill insects. Choose a repellent containing DEET (*N, N*-diethyl-*m*-toluamide), IR3535® (3-[*N*-acetyl-*N*-butyl]-aminopropionic acid ethyl ester) or Bayrepel® (1-piperidinecarboxylic acid, 2-(2-hydroxyethyl)- 1-methylpropylester). Insect repellents should be applied to provide protection at times when insects are biting. Care must be taken to avoid contact with mucous membranes. Insect repellents should not be sprayed on the face or applied to the eyelids or lips. Always wash the hands after applying the repellent. Insect repellents should not be applied to sensitive, sunburned or damaged skin or deep skin folds. Repeated applications may be required every 3–4 hours, especially in hot and humid climates. When the product is applied to clothes, the repellent effect lasts longer. Repellents should be used in strict accordance with the manufacturers' instructions and the dosage must not be exceeded, especially for young children and pregnant women.

Mosquito nets are excellent means of personal protection while sleeping. Nets can be used either with or without insecticide treatment. However, treated nets are much more effective. Pretreated nets may be commercially available. Nets should be strong and with a mesh size no larger than 1.5 mm. The net should be tucked in under the mattress, ensuring first that it is not torn and that there are no mosquitoes inside. Nets for hammocks are available, as are nets for cots and small beds.

Mosquito coils are the best known example of insecticide vaporizer, usually with a synthetic pyrethroid as the active ingredient. One coil serves a normal bedroom through the night, unless the room is particularly draughty. A more sophisticated version, which requires electricity, is an insecticide mat that is placed on an electrically heated grid, causing the insecticide to vaporize. Such devices can also be used during daytime if necessary.

Aerosol sprays intended to kill flying insects are effective for quick knockdown and killing. Indoor sleeping areas should be sprayed before bedtime. Treating a room with an insecticide spray will help to free it from insects, but the effect may be short-lived. Spraying combined with the use of a coil, a vaporizer or a mosquito net is recommended. Aerosol sprays intended for crawling insects (e.g. cockroaches and ants) should be sprayed on surfaces where these insects walk.

Protective clothing can help at times of the day when vectors are active. The thickness of the material is critical. Exposed skin should be treated with a repellent. Insect repellent applied to clothing is effective for longer than it may be on the skin. Extra protection is provided by treating clothing with permethrin or etofenprox, to prevent mosquitoes from biting through clothing. Label instructions should be followed to avoid damage to certain fabrics. In tick- and flea-infested areas, feet should be protected by appropriate footwear and by tucking long trousers into the socks. Such measures are further enhanced by application of repellents to the clothing.

Travellers camping in tents should use a combination of mosquito coils, repellents and screens. The mesh size of tent screens often exceeds 1.5 mm, so that special mosquito screens have to be deployed.

Screening of windows, doors and eaves reduces exposure to flying insects. Accommodation with these features should be sought where available.

Air-conditioning is a highly effective means of keeping mosquitoes and other insects out of a room. In air-conditioned hotels, other precautions are not necessary indoors.

Avoid contact with freshwater bodies such as lakes, irrigation ditches and slow-running streams in areas where schistosomiasis occurs.

Table 3.1 **Principal disease vectors and the diseases they transmit**[a]

Vectors	Main diseases transmitted
Aquatic snails	Schistosomiasis (bilharziasis)
Blackflies	River blindness (onchocerciasis)
Fleas	Plague (transmitted by fleas from rats to humans)
Mosquitoes	
Aedes	Dengue fever
	Rift Valley fever
	Yellow fever
	Chikungunya
Anopheles	Lymphatic filariasis
	Malaria
Culex	Japanese encephalitis
	Lymphatic filariasis
	West Nile fever
Sandflies	Leishmaniasis
	Sandfly fever (*Phlebotomus* fever)
Ticks	Crimean–Congo haemorrhagic fever
	Lyme disease
	Relapsing fever (borreliosis)
	Rickettsial diseases including spotted fevers and Q fever
	Tick-borne encephalitis
	Tularaemia
Triatomine bugs	Chagas disease (American trypanosomiasis)
Tsetse flies	Sleeping sickness (African trypanosomiasis)

[a] Based on extensive research, there is absolutely no evidence that HIV infection can be transmitted by insects.

Further reading

Bites and stings due to terrestrial and aquatic animals in Europe: http://www.who.int/wer/pdf/2001/wer7638.pdf

Foodborne disease: a focus on health education. Geneva, World Health Organization, 2000. (See annex for comprehensive information on 31 foodborne diseases caused by bacteria, viruses and parasites.)

Hackett PH, Roach RC. High-altitude illness. *New England Journal of Medicine*, 2001, 345: 107–114.

Preventing travellers' diarrhoea: how to make drinking-water safe: http://www.who.int/water_sanitation_health/hygiene/envsan/travel/en/index.html

Rozendaal J. *Vector control: methods for use by individuals and communities.* Geneva, World Health Organization, 1997.

Vectors of disease, Part I: http://www.who.int/wer/pdf/2001/wer7625.pdf

Vectors of disease, Part II: http://www.who.int/wer/pdf/2001/wer7626.pdf

WHO advice on sun protection: http://www.who.int/uv/en

WHO guide on safe food for travellers: http://www.who.int/fsf/brochure/trvl1.htm

WHO guidelines for safe recreational waters:
Volume 1: Coastal and fresh waters
http://www.who.int/water_sanitation_health/bathing/srwe1execsum/en/index3.html
Volume 2: Swimming pools and similar recreational-water environments
http://www.who.int/water_sanitation_health/bathing/bathing2/en/

CHAPTER 4

Injuries and violence

Travellers are more likely to be killed or injured through violence or unintentional injuries than to be struck down by an exotic infectious disease. Traffic collisions are the most frequent cause of death among travellers. Road traffic collisions and violence are significant risks in many countries, particularly developing countries, where skilled medical care may not be readily available. Injuries also occur in other settings, particularly in recreational waters in association with swimming, diving, sailing and other activities. Travellers can reduce the possibility of incurring these risks through awareness of the dangers and by taking the appropriate precautions.

Road traffic injuries

Worldwide, an estimated 1.2 million people are killed each year in road traffic crashes and as many as 50 million more are injured. Projections indicate that these figures will increase by about 65% over the next 20 years unless there is new commitment to prevention.

In many developing countries traffic laws are limited or are inadequately enforced. Often the traffic mix is more complex than that in developed countries and involves two- three- and four-wheeled vehicles, animal-drawn vehicles and other conveyances, plus pedestrians, all sharing the same road space. The roads may be poorly constructed and maintained, road signs and lighting inadequate and driving habits poor. Travellers, both drivers and pedestrians, should be extremely attentive and careful on the roads.

There are a number of practical precautions that travellers can take to reduce the risk of being involved in, or becoming the victim of, a road traffic crash.

Precautions
- Have full insurance cover for medical treatment of both illness and injuries.
- Carry an international driving licence as well as your national driving licence.

- Obtain information on the regulations governing traffic and vehicle mainte-nance, and on the state of the roads, in the countries to be visited.

- Before renting a car check the state of the tyres, seat belts, spare wheels, lights, brakes, etc.

- Know the informal rules of the road; in some countries, for example, it is cus-tomary to sound the horn or flash the headlights before overtaking.

- Be particularly vigilant in a country where the traffic drives on the opposite side of the road to that used in your country of residence.

- Do not drive on unfamiliar and unlit roads.

- Do not use a moped, motorcycle, bicycle or tricycle.

- Do not drive after drinking alcohol.

- Drive within the speed limit at all times.

- Always wear a seat belt where these are available.

- Beware of wandering animals.

Injuries in recreational waters

Recreational waters include coastal waters, freshwater lakes and rivers, swimming pools and spas. The hazards associated with recreational waters can be minimized by safe behaviour and simple precautions.

The most important health hazards in recreational waters are drowning and impact injuries, particularly head and spinal injuries. It is estimated that almost 400 000 deaths are caused by drowning every year. In addition, many more cases of "non-fatal drowning" occur, often with life-long effects on health.

Drowning may occur when a person is caught in a tide or rip current, is trapped by rising tides, falls overboard from a boat, becomes caught in submerged obstacles, or falls asleep on an inflatable mattress and is carried out to sea. In swimming pools and spas, drowning or near-drowning and other injuries may occur close to outlets where suction is strong enough to catch body parts or hair so that the head is trapped under water. Drowning in swimming pools may be related to slip–trip–fall incidents leading to loss of consciousness on impact. If the water is not clear it may be difficult to see submerged swimmers or obstacles, increasing the chances of an accident in the water.

Children can drown in a very short time and in relatively small amounts of water. The factor that contributes most frequently to children drowning is lack of adult supervision. Children in or near water should be constantly supervised by adults.

Drowning is also a hazard for those wading and fishing. Falling in cold water, particularly when wearing heavy clothing, may result in drowning as swimming ability is hampered.

Impact injuries are usually the result of diving accidents, particularly diving into shallow water and/or hitting underwater obstructions. Water may appear to be deeper than it is. Impact of the head on a hard surface may cause head and/or spinal injuries. Spinal injuries may result in various degrees of paraplegia or quadriplegia. Head injuries may cause concussion and loss of memory and/or motor skills.

Drowning and impact injuries in adults are frequently associated with alcohol consumption, which impairs judgement and the ability to react effectively.

A detached retina, which can result in blindness or near-blindness, may be caused by jumping into water or jumping onto other people in the water.

Precautions

- Adopt safe behaviour in all recreational waters: use life jackets where appropriate, pay attention to tides and currents, and avoid outlets in spas and swimming pools.
- Ensure constant adult supervision of children in or near recreational waters, including small volumes of water.
- Avoid consumption of alcohol before any activity in or near water.
- Check the depth of the water carefully before diving, and avoid diving or jumping into murky water as submerged swimmers or objects may not be visible.
- Do not jump into water or jump onto others in the water.

Violence

Violence is a significant risk in many developing countries. Criminals often target tourists and business travellers, particularly in countries where crime levels are high. However, some sensible precautions may reduce this risk.

Precautions

- Be alert to the possibility of muggings during the day as well as at night.
- Keep jewellery, cameras and other items of value out of sight and do not carry large sums of money on your person.

- Avoid isolated beaches and other remote areas.
- Avoid overcrowded trains, buses and minibus taxis.
- Use taxis from authorized ranks only.
- Avoid driving at night and never travel alone.
- Keep car doors locked and windows shut.
- Be particularly alert when waiting at traffic lights.
- Park in well-lit areas and do not pick up strangers.
- Employ the services of a local guide/interpreter or local driver when travelling to remote areas.
- Vehicle hijacking is a recognized risk in a number of countries. If stopped by armed robbers, make no attempt to resist and keep hands where the attackers can see them at all times.

Further reading

WHO information on violence and injury prevention: http://www.who.int/violence_injury_prevention/en

CHAPTER 5

Infectious diseases of potential risk for travellers

Depending on the travel destination, travellers may be exposed to a number of infectious diseases; exposure depends on the presence of infectious agents in the area to be visited. The risk of becoming infected will vary according to the purpose of the trip and the itinerary within the area, the standards of accommodation, hygiene and sanitation, as well as the behaviour of the traveller. In some instances, disease can be prevented by vaccination, but there are some infectious diseases, including some of the most important and most dangerous, for which no vaccines exist.

General precautions can greatly reduce the risk of exposure to infectious agents and should always be taken for visits to any destination where there is a significant risk of exposure. These precautions should be taken regardless of whether any vaccinations or medication have been administered.

Modes of transmission and general precautions

The modes of transmission for different infectious diseases and the corresponding general precautions are outlined in the following paragraphs.

Foodborne and waterborne diseases

Food- and waterborne diseases are transmitted by consumption of contaminated food and drink. The risk of infection is reduced by taking hygienic precautions with all food, drink and drinking-water consumed when travelling and by avoiding direct contact with polluted recreational waters (see Chapter 3). Examples of diseases transmitted by food and water are hepatitis A, typhoid fever and cholera.

Vector-borne diseases

A number of particularly serious infections are transmitted by insects and other vectors such as ticks. The risk of infection can be reduced by taking precautions to avoid insect bites and contact with other vectors in places where infection is likely to be present (see Chapter 3). Examples of vector-borne diseases are malaria, yellow fever, dengue and tick-borne encephalitis.

Zoonoses (diseases transmitted from animals)

Zoonoses include many infections that can be transmitted to humans through animal bites or contact with contaminated body fluids or faeces from animals, or by consumption of foods of animal origin, particularly meat and milk products. The risk of infection can be reduced by avoiding close contact with any animals—including wild, captive and domestic animals—in places where infection is likely to be present. Particular care should be taken to prevent children from approaching and handling animals. Examples of zoonoses are rabies, brucellosis, leptospirosis and certain viral haemorrhagic fevers.

Sexually transmitted diseases

Sexually transmitted diseases are passed from person to person through unsafe sexual practices. The risk of infection can be reduced by avoiding casual and unprotected sexual intercourse, and by use of condoms. Examples of sexually transmitted diseases are hepatitis B, HIV/AIDS and syphilis.

Bloodborne diseases

Bloodborne diseases are transmitted by direct contact with infected blood or other body fluids. The risk of infection can be reduced by avoiding direct contact with blood and body fluids, by avoiding the use of potentially contaminated needles and syringes for injection or any other medical or cosmetic procedure that penetrates the skin (including acupuncture, piercing and tattooing), and by avoiding transfusion of unsafe blood (see Chapter 8). Examples of bloodborne diseases are hepatitis B and C, HIV/AIDS and malaria.

Airborne diseases

Airborne diseases are transmitted from person to person by aerosol and droplets from the nose and mouth. The risk of infection can be reduced by avoiding close contact with people in crowded and enclosed places. Examples of airborne diseases are influenza, measles and tuberculosis.

Diseases transmitted from soil

Soil-transmitted diseases include those caused by dormant forms (spores) of infectious agents, which can cause infection by contact with broken skin (minor cuts, scratches, etc.). The risk of infection can be reduced by protecting the skin from direct contact with soil in places where soil-transmitted infections are likely to be present. Examples of bacterial diseases transmitted from soil are anthrax and tetanus. Certain intestinal parasitic infections, such as ascariasis and trichuriasis, are transmitted via soil and infection may result from consumption of soil-contaminated vegetables.

Specific infectious diseases involving potential health risks for travellers

The main infectious diseases to which travellers may be exposed, and precautions for each, are detailed on the following pages. Information on malaria, the most important infectious disease threat for travellers, is provided in Chapter 7. Other infectious diseases that affect travellers only rarely are not described in this book. The infectious diseases described in this chapter have been selected on the basis of the following criteria:

— diseases that have a sufficiently high global or regional prevalence to constitute a significant risk for travellers;
— diseases that are severe and life-threatening, even though the risk of exposure may be low for most travellers;
— diseases for which the perceived risk may be much greater than the real risk, and which may therefore cause anxiety to travellers;
— diseases that involve a public health risk due to transmission of infection to others by the infected traveller.

Information about available vaccines and indications for their use by travellers is provided in Chapter 6. Advice concerning the diseases for which vaccination is routinely administered in childhood, i.e. diphtheria, measles, mumps and rubella, pertussis, poliomyelitis and tetanus, and the use of the corresponding vaccines later in life and for travel, is also given in Chapter 6. These diseases are not included in this chapter.

The most common infectious illness to affect travellers, namely travellers' diarrhoea, is covered in Chapter 3. Because travellers' diarrhoea can be caused by many different foodborne and waterborne infectious agents, for which treatment and precautions are essentially the same, the illness is not included with the specific infectious diseases.

Some of the diseases included in this chapter, such as brucellosis, HIV/AIDS, leishmaniasis and tuberculosis, have prolonged and variable incubation periods. Clinical manifestations of these diseases may appear long after the return from travel, so that the link with the travel destination where the infection was acquired may not be readily apparent.

AVIAN INFLUENZA

Cause	Avian influenza A virus H5N1, and sometimes other avian influenza subtypes (H7, H9)
Transmission	Human infections with avian influenza H5N1 occur through bird-to-human, possibly environment-to-human, and limited, non-sustained human-to-human transmission. Direct contact with infected poultry, or surfaces and objects contaminated by their droppings, is the main route of spread to humans. Exposure risk is considered highest during slaughter, de-feathering, butchering, and preparation of poultry for cooking. There is no evidence that properly cooked poultry or poultry products can be a source of infection.
Nature of disease	Presenting symptoms are usually fever and an influenza-like illness (malaise, myalgia, cough, sore throat). Diarrhoea and other gastrointestinal symptoms are common. Sputum production is variable and sometimes bloody. Almost all patients have clinically apparent pneumonia with radiographic infiltrates of varying patterns. Encephalopathy, multi-organ failure and sepsis-like syndromes occur. The fatality rate among hospitalized patients with confirmed H5N1 infection has been high (over 50%), most commonly as a result of respiratory failure due to progressive pneumonia and acute respiratory distress syndrome.
Geographical distribution	Extensive outbreaks have occurred in poultry in parts of Asia, the Middle East, Europe and Africa since 2003, but only sporadic human infections have occurred to date. Continued exposure of humans to avian H5N1 viruses increases the likelihood that the virus will acquire the necessary characteristics for efficient and sustained human-to-human transmission through either gradual genetic mutation or re-assortment with a human influenza A virus. Between November 2003 and mid-October 2006, 256 human cases of proven H5N1 infection were reported to WHO from 10 countries in South-East and central Asia, Europe, Africa and the Middle East.
Risk for travellers	H5N1 avian influenza is primarily a disease in birds. The virus does not easily cross the species barrier to infect humans. The risk of infection depends on proximity to infected birds.
Prophylaxis	No human H5 vaccine is commercially available at present. Neuraminidase inhibitors (oseltamivir, zanamivir) are inhibitory for the virus and are recommended for post-exposure prophylaxis in certain exposed persons (http://www.who.int/csr/disease/avian_influenza/guidelines/pharmamanagement/en/index.html). At present WHO does not recommend pre-exposure prophylaxis for travellers but advice may change depending on new findings.
Precautions	Travellers should avoid contact with high-risk environments in affected countries such as live animal markets and poultry farms, any free-ranging or caged poultry, or surfaces that might be contaminated by poultry droppings. Travellers in affected countries should avoid contact with dead migratory birds or wild birds showing signs of disease. Hand hygiene with frequent washing or use of alcohol rubs is recommended. If exposure to persons with suspected H5N1 illness or severe, unexplained respiratory illness occurs, travellers should urgently consult health professionals. Travellers should contact their local health providers or national health authorities for supplementary information.

ANTHRAX

Cause	*Bacillus anthracis* bacteria.
Transmission	Cutaneous infection, the most frequent clinical form of anthrax, occurs through contact with contaminated products from infected animals (mainly cattle, goats, sheep), such as leather or woollen goods, or through contact with soil containing anthrax spores.
Nature of the disease	A disease of herbivorous animals that occasionally causes acute infection in humans, usually involving the skin, as a result of contact with contaminated tissues or products from infected animals, or with anthrax spores in soil. Untreated infections may spread to regional lymph nodes and to the bloodstream, and may be fatal.
Geographical distribution	Sporadic cases occur in animals worldwide; there are occasional outbreaks in central Asia and Africa.
Risk for travellers	Very low for most travellers.
Prophylaxis	None. (A vaccine is available for people at high risk because of occupational exposure to *B. anthracis*; it is not commercially available in most countries.)
Precautions	Avoid direct contact with soil and with products of animal origin, such as souvenirs made from animal skins.

BRUCELLOSIS

Cause	Several species of *Brucella* bacteria.
Transmission	Brucellosis is primarily a disease of animals. Infection occurs from cattle (*Brucella abortus*), dogs (*B. canis*), pigs (*B. suis*), or sheep and goats (*B. melitensis*), usually by direct contact with infected animals or by consumption of unpasteurized (raw) milk or cheese.
Nature of the disease	A generalized infection with insidious onset, causing continuous or intermittent fever and malaise, which may last for months if not treated adequately. Relapse is common after treatment.
Geographical distribution	Worldwide, in animals. It is most common in developing countries and the Mediterranean region.
Risk for travellers	Low for most travellers. Those visiting rural and agricultural areas may be at greater risk. There is also a risk in places where unpasteurized milk products are sold near tourist centres.
Prophylaxis	None.
Precautions	Avoid consumption of unpasteurized milk and milk products and direct contact with animals, particularly cattle, goats and sheep.

CHIKUNGUNYA

Cause	Chikungunya virus – an Alphavirus (family Togaviridae).
Transmission	Chikungunya is transmitted by mosquitoes, including many *Aedes* species which bite during daylight hours. Two important vectors in Asia are *Aedes aegypti* and *Aedes albopictus*, both of which also transmit dengue virus. There is no direct person-to-person transmission. The virus has been isolated from monkeys in Africa.
Nature of the disease	Chikungunya is an acute febrile illness with sudden onset of fever and joint pains, particularly affecting the hands, wrists, ankles and feet. There may be severe chills, leukopenia and often a rash. Generalized myalgia is also common. The name chikungunya derives from Swahili and means "that which bends up". Most patients recover after a few days but in some cases the joint pains may persist for week, months or even longer. Chikungunya may also be asymptomatic.
Geographical distribution	Chikungunya occurs in sub-Saharan Africa, south-east Asia and tropical areas of the Indian subcontinent, as well as islands in the south-west Indian Ocean.
Risk for travellers	There is a risk for travellers in areas where chikungunya is endemic and in areas affected by epidemics.
Prophylaxis	None.
Precautions	Travellers should take precautions to avoid mosquito bites both during the day and at night in areas where chikungunya occurs.

CHOLERA

Cause	*Vibrio cholerae* bacteria, serogroups O1 and O139.
Transmission	Infection occurs through ingestion of food or water contaminated directly or indirectly by faeces or vomitus of infected persons. Cholera affects only humans; there is no insect vector or animal reservoir host.
Nature of the disease	An acute enteric disease varying in severity. Most infections are asymptomatic (i.e. do not cause any illness). In mild cases, diarrhoea occurs without other symptoms. In severe cases, there is sudden onset of profuse watery diarrhoea with nausea and vomiting and rapid development of dehydration. In severe untreated cases, death may occur within a few hours due to dehydration leading to circulatory collapse.
Geographical distribution	Cholera occurs mainly in poor countries with inadequate sanitation and lack of clean drinking-water and in war-torn countries where the infrastructure may have broken down. Many developing countries are affected, particularly those in Africa and Asia, and to a lesser extent those in central and south America (see map).
Risk for travellers	Very low for most travellers, even in countries where cholera epidemics occur. Humanitarian relief workers in disaster areas and refugee camps are at risk.

Prophylaxis	Cholera vaccines for use by travellers and those in occupational risk groups are available in some countries (see Chapter 6).
Precautions	As for other diarrhoeal diseases. All precautions should be taken to avoid consumption of potentially contaminated food, drink and drinking-water. Oral rehydration salts should be carried to combat dehydration in case of severe diarrhoea (see Chapter 3).

DENGUE

Cause	The dengue virus – a flavivirus of which there are four serotypes.
Transmission	Dengue is mostly transmitted by the *Aedes aegypti* mosquito, which bites during daylight hours. There is no direct person-to-person transmission. Monkeys act as a reservoir host in South-East Asia and West Africa.
Nature of the disease	Dengue occurs in three main clinical forms: ■ Dengue fever is an acute febrile illness with sudden onset of fever, followed by development of generalized symptoms and sometimes a macular skin rash. It is known as "breakbone fever" because of severe muscular pains. The fever may be biphasic (i.e. two separate episodes or waves of fever). Most patients recover after a few days. ■ Dengue haemorrhagic fever has an acute onset of fever followed by other symptoms resulting from thrombocytopenia, increased vascular permeability and haemorrhagic manifestations. ■ Dengue shock syndrome supervenes in a small proportion of cases. Severe hypotension develops, requiring urgent medical treatment to correct hypovolaemia. Without appropriate treatment, 40–50% of cases are fatal; with timely therapy, the mortality rate is 1% or less.
Geographical distribution	Dengue is widespread in tropical and subtropical regions of central and south America and south and south-east Asia and also occurs in Africa (see map). The risk is lower at altitudes above 1000 metres.
Risk for travellers	There is a significant risk for travellers in areas where dengue is endemic and in areas affected by epidemics of dengue.
Prophylaxis	None.
Precautions	Travellers should take precautions to avoid mosquito bites both during the day and at night in areas where dengue occurs.

FILARIASIS

Cause	The parasitic diseases covered by the term filariasis are caused by nematodes (roundworms) of the family Filarioidea. Diseases in this group include lymphatic filariasis and onchocerciasis (river blindness).
Transmission	Lymphatic filariasis is transmitted through the bite of infected mosquitoes, which introduce larval forms of the nematode during a blood meal. Onchocerciasis is transmitted through the bite of infected blackflies.

Nature of the disease	■ Lymphatic filariasis is a chronic parasitic disease in which adult filaria inhabit the lymphatic vessels, discharging microfilaria into the blood stream. Typical manifestations in symptomatic cases include filarial fever, lymphadenitis and retrograde lymphangitis followed by chronic manifestations like lymphoedema, hydrocele, chyluria and in rare instances renal damage.
	■ Onchocerciasis is a chronic parasitic disease occurring mainly in sub-Saharan west Africa in which adult worms are found in fibrous nodules under the skin. They discharge microfilaria, which migrate through the skin causing dermatitis, and reach the eye causing damage that results in blindness.
Geographical distribution	Lymphatic filariasis occurs throughout sub-Saharan Africa and in much of South-East Asia, in the Pacific islands and in smaller foci in south America. Onchocerciasis occurs mainly in western and central Africa, also in central and south America.
Risk for travellers	Generally low, unless travel involves extensive exposure to the vectors in endemic areas.
Prophylaxis	None.
Precautions	Avoid exposure to the bites of mosquitoes and/or blackflies in endemic areas.

GIARDIASIS

Cause	The protozoan parasite *Giardia intestinalis*, also known as *G. lamblia* and *G. duodenalis*.
Transmission	Infection usually occurs through ingestion of *G. intestinalis* cysts in water (including both unfiltered drinking-water and recreational waters) contaminated by the faeces of infected humans or animals.
Nature of the disease	Many infections are asymptomatic. When symptoms occur, they are mainly intestinal, characterized by chronic diarrhoea (watery initially, then loose greasy stools), abdominal cramps, bloating, fatigue and weight loss.
Geographical distribution	Worldwide.
Risk for travellers	Significant risk for travellers in contact with recreational waters used by wildlife or with unfiltered water in swimming pools.
Prophylaxis	None.
Precautions	Avoid ingesting any potentially contaminated (i.e. unfiltered) drinking-water or recreational water.

HAEMOPHILUS MENINGITIS

Cause	*Haemophilus influenzae* type b (Hib) bacteria.
Transmission	Direct contact with infected persons (usually children).
Nature of the disease	Hib causes meningitis in infants and young children; it may also cause epiglottitis, osteomyelitis, pneumonia, sepsis and septic arthritis.

Geographical distribution	Worldwide. Hib disease is most common in countries where vaccination against Hib is not practised. It has almost disappeared in countries where routine childhood vaccination is carried out.
Risk for travellers	A risk for unvaccinated children visiting countries where Hib vaccination is not practised and where infection is therefore likely to be more common.
Prophylaxis	Vaccination of children (see Chapter 6).
Precautions	None.

HAEMORRHAGIC FEVERS

Haemorrhagic fevers are viral infections; important examples are Crimean–Congo haemorrhagic fever (CCHF), dengue, Ebola and Marburg haemorrhagic fevers, Lassa fever, Rift Valley fever (RVF) and yellow fever.

Dengue and yellow fever are described separately.

Cause	Viruses belonging to several families. Most haemorrhagic fevers, including dengue and yellow fever, are caused by flaviviruses; Ebola and Marburg are caused by filoviruses, CCHF by a bunyavirus, Lassa fever by an arenavirus, and RVF by a phlebovirus.
Transmission	Most viruses that cause haemorrhagic fevers are transmitted by mosquitoes. However, no insect vector has so far been identified for Ebola or Marburg viruses: these viruses are acquired by direct contact with the body fluids or secretions of infected patients. CCHF is transmitted by ticks. Lassa fever virus is carried by rodents and transmitted by excreta, either as aerosol or by direct contact. RVF can be acquired either by mosquito bite or by direct contact with blood or tissues of infected animals (mainly sheep), including consumption of unpasteurized milk.
Nature of the diseases	The haemorrhagic fevers are severe acute viral infections, usually with sudden onset of fever, malaise, headache and myalgia followed by pharyngitis, vomiting, diarrhoea, skin rash and haemorrhagic manifestations. The outcome is fatal in a high proportion of cases (over 50%).
Geographical distribution	Diseases in this group occur widely in tropical and subtropical regions. Ebola and Marburg haemorrhagic fevers and Lassa fever occur in sub-Saharan Africa. CCHF occurs in the steppe regions of central Asia and in central Europe, as well as in tropical and southern Africa. RVF occurs in Africa and has recently spread to Saudi Arabia. Other viral haemorrhagic fevers occur in central and south America.
Risk for travellers	Very low for most travellers. However, travellers visiting rural or forest areas may be exposed to infection.
Prophylaxis	None (except for yellow fever).
Precautions	Avoid exposure to mosquitoes and ticks and contact with rodents.

HANTAVIRUS DISEASES

Hantavirus diseases are viral infections; important examples are haemorrhagic fever with renal syndrome (HFRS) and hantavirus pulmonary syndrome (HPS).

Cause	Hantaviruses, which belong to the family of bunyaviruses.
Transmission	Hantaviruses are carried by various species of rodents. Infection occurs through direct contact with the faeces, saliva or urine of infected rodents or by inhalation of the virus by aerosol transmission from rodent excreta.
Nature of the diseases	Acute viral diseases in which vascular endothelium is damaged, leading to increased vascular permeability, hypotension, haemorrhagic manifestations and shock. Impaired renal function with oliguria is characteristic of HFRS. Respiratory distress due to pulmonary oedema occurs in HPS. The outcome is fatal in up to 15% of HFRS cases and up to 50% of HPS cases.
Geographical distribution	Worldwide, in rodents.
Risk for travellers	Very low for most travellers. However, travellers may be at risk in any environment where rodents are present in large numbers and contact may occur.
Prophylaxis	None.
Precautions	Avoid exposure to rodents and their excreta. Adventure travellers, back-packers, campers and travellers with occupational exposure to rodents in areas endemic for hantaviruses should take precautions to exclude rodents from tents or other accommodation and to protect all food from contamination by rodents.

HEPATITIS A

Cause	Hepatitis A virus, a member of the picornavirus family.
Transmission	The virus is acquired directly from infected persons by the faecal–oral route or by close contact, or by consumption of contaminated food or drinking-water. There is no insect vector or animal reservoir (although some non-human primates are sometimes infected).
Nature of the disease	An acute viral hepatitis with abrupt onset of fever, malaise, nausea and abdominal discomfort, followed by the development of jaundice a few days later. Infection in very young children is usually mild or asymptomatic; older children are at risk of symptomatic disease. The disease is more severe in adults, with illness lasting several weeks and recovery taking several months; case-fatality is greater than 2% for those over 40 years of age and 4% for those over 60.
Geographical distribution	Worldwide, but most common where sanitary conditions are poor and the safety of drinking-water is not well controlled (see map).
Risk for travellers	Non-immune travellers to developing countries are at significant risk of infection. The risk is particularly high for travellers exposed to poor conditions of hygiene, sanitation and drinking-water control.
Prophylaxis	Vaccination (see Chapter 6).

Precautions	Travellers who are non-immune to hepatitis A (i.e. have never had the disease and have not been vaccinated) should take particular care to avoid potentially contaminated food and water.

HEPATITIS B

Cause	Hepatitis B virus (HBV), belonging to the Hepadnaviridae.
Transmission	Infection is transmitted from person to person by contact with infected body fluids. Sexual contact is an important mode of transmission, but infection is also transmitted by transfusion of contaminated blood or blood products, or by use of contaminated needles or syringes for injections. There is also a potential risk of transmission through other skin-penetrating procedures including acupuncture, piercing and tattooing. Perinatal transmission may occur from mother to baby. There is no insect vector or animal reservoir.
Nature of the disease	Many HBV infections are asymptomatic or cause mild symptoms, which are often unrecognized in adults. When clinical hepatitis results from infection, it has a gradual onset, with anorexia, abdominal discomfort, nausea, vomiting, arthralgia and rash, followed by the development of jaundice in some cases. In adults, about 1% of cases are fatal. Chronic HBV infection persists in a proportion of adults, some of whom later develop cirrhosis and/or liver cancer.
Geographical distribution	Worldwide, but with differing levels of endemicity. In north America, Australia, northern and western Europe and New Zealand, prevalence of chronic HBV infection is relatively low (less than 2% of the general population) (see map).
Risk for travellers	Negligible for those vaccinated against hepatitis B. Unvaccinated travellers are at risk if they have unprotected sex or use contaminated needles or syringes for injection, acupuncture, piercing or tattooing. An accident or medical emergency requiring blood transfusion may result in infection if the blood has not been screened for HBV. Travellers engaged in humanitarian relief activities may be exposed to infected blood or other body fluids in health care settings (see box).
Prophylaxis	Vaccination (see Chapter 6).
Precautions	Adopt safe sexual practices and avoid the use of any potentially contaminated instruments for injection or other skin-piercing activity.

HEPATITIS C

Cause	Hepatitis C virus (HCV), which is a flavivirus.
Transmission	The virus is acquired through person-to-person transmission by parenteral routes. Before screening for HCV became available, infection was mainly transmitted by transfusion of contaminated blood or blood products. Nowadays transmission frequently occurs through use of contaminated needles, syringes and other instruments used for injections and other skin-piercing procedures. Sexual transmission of hepatitis C occurs rarely. There is no insect vector or animal reservoir for HCV.

Nature of the disease	Most HCV infections are asymptomatic. In cases where infection leads to clinical hepatitis, the onset of symptoms is usually gradual, with anorexia, abdominal discomfort, nausea and vomiting, followed by the development of jaundice in some cases (less commonly than in hepatitis B). Most clinically affected patients will develop a long-lasting chronic infection, which may lead to cirrhosis and/or liver cancer.
Geographical distribution	Worldwide, with regional differences in levels of prevalence (see map).
Risk for travellers	Travellers are at risk if they practise unsafe behaviour involving the use of contaminated needles or syringes for injection, acupuncture, piercing or tattooing. An accident or medical emergency requiring blood transfusion may result in infection if the blood has not been screened for HCV. Travellers engaged in humanitarian relief activities may be exposed to infected blood or other body fluids in health care settings.
Prophylaxis	None.
Precautions	Adopt safe sexual practices and avoid the use of any potentially contaminated instruments for injection or other skin-piercing activity.

HEPATITIS E

Cause	Hepatitis E virus, which has not yet been definitively classified (formerly classified as a member of the Caliciviridae).
Transmission	Hepatitis E is a waterborne disease usually acquired from contaminated drinking-water. Direct faecal–oral transmission from person to person is also possible. There is no insect vector. It is suspected, but not proved, that hepatitis E may have a domestic animal reservoir host, such as pigs.
Nature of the disease	The clinical features and course of the disease are generally similar to those of hepatitis A. As with hepatitis A, there is no chronic phase. Young adults are most commonly affected. In pregnant women there is an important difference between hepatitis E and hepatitis A: during the third trimester of pregnancy, hepatitis E takes a much more severe form with a case-fatality rate reaching 20%.
Geographical distribution	Worldwide. Most cases, both sporadic and epidemic, occur in countries with poor standards of hygiene and sanitation.
Risk for travellers	Travellers to developing countries may be at risk when exposed to poor conditions of sanitation and drinking-water control.
Prophylaxis	None.
Precautions	Travellers should follow the general conditions for avoiding potentially contaminated food and drinking-water (see Chapter 3).

HIV/AIDS AND OTHER SEXUALLY TRANSMITTED INFECTIONS

The most important sexually transmitted diseases and infectious agents are:

HIV/AIDS	human immunodeficiency virus
hepatitis B	hepatitis B virus
syphilis	*Treponema pallidum*

gonorrhoea	*Neisseria gonorrhoeae*
chlamydial infections	*Chlamydia trachomatis*
trichomoniasis	*Trichomonas vaginalis*
chancroid	*Haemophilus ducreyi*
genital herpes	herpes simplex virus (human (alpha) herpesvirus 2)
genital warts	human papillomavirus

Travel restrictions

Some countries have adopted entry and visa restrictions for people with HIV/AIDS. Travellers who are infected with HIV should consult their personal physician for a detailed assessment and advice before travel. WHO has taken the position that there is no public health justification for entry restrictions that discriminate solely on the basis of a person's HIV status.

Transmission	Infection occurs during unprotected sexual intercourse. Hepatitis B, HIV and syphilis may also be transmitted in contaminated blood and blood products, by contaminated syringes and needles used for injection, and potentially by unsterilized instruments used for acupuncture, piercing and tattooing.
Nature of the diseases	Most of the clinical manifestations are included in the following syndromes: genital ulcer, pelvic inflammatory disease, urethral discharge and vaginal discharge. However, many infections are asymptomatic.
	Sexually transmitted infections are a major cause of acute illness, infertility, long-term disability and death, with severe medical and psychological consequences for millions of men, women and children.
	Apart from being serious diseases in their own right, sexually transmitted infections increase the risk of HIV infection. The presence of an untreated disease (ulcerative or non-ulcerative) can increase by a factor of up to 10 the risk of becoming infected with HIV and transmitting the infection. On the other hand, early diagnosis and improved management of other sexually transmitted infections can reduce the incidence of HIV infection by up to 40%. Prevention and treatment of all sexually transmitted infections are therefore important for the prevention of HIV infection.
Geographical distribution	Worldwide (see map). The regional differences in the prevalence of HIV infection are shown on the map. Sexually transmitted infections have been known since ancient times; they remain a major public health problem, which was compounded by the appearance of HIV/AIDS around 1980. An estimated 340 million episodes of curable sexually transmitted infections (chlamydial infections, gonorrhoea, syphilis, trichomoniasis) occur throughout the world every year. Viral infections, which are more difficult to treat, are also very common in many populations. Genital herpes is becoming a major cause of genital ulcer, and subtypes of the human papillomavirus are associated with cervical cancer.
Risk for travellers	For some travellers there may be an increased risk of infection. Lack of information about risk and preventive measures and the fact that travel and tourism enhance the probability of having sex with casual partners increase the risk of exposure to sexually transmitted infections. In some developed countries, a large proportion of sexually transmitted infections now occur as a result of unprotected sexual intercourse during international travel.
	In addition to transmission through sexual intercourse (both heterosexual and homosexual – anal, vaginal or oral), some of these infections can be passed

on from an infected mother to her unborn or newborn baby. Hepatitis B, HIV and syphilis are also transmitted through transfusion of contaminated blood or blood products and the use of contaminated needles.

There is no risk of acquiring any sexually transmitted infection from casual day-to-day contact at home, at work or socially. People run no risk of infection when sharing any means of communal transport (e.g. aircraft, boat, bus, car, train) with infected individuals. There is no evidence that HIV or other sexually transmitted infections can be acquired from insect bites.

Prophylaxis

Vaccination against hepatitis B (see Chapter 6). Preventive vaccines against oncogenic types of human papillomavirus show great promise and will soon be available. No prophylaxis is available for any of the other sexually transmitted diseases. For post-exposure prophylaxis see Chapter 8.

Precautions

Male or female condoms, when used properly and consistently, have proved to be effective in preventing the transmission of HIV and other sexually transmitted infections, and for reducing the risk of unwanted pregnancy. Latex rubber condoms are relatively inexpensive, are highly reliable and have virtually no side-effects. The transmission of HIV and other infections during sexual intercourse can be effectively prevented when high-quality condoms are used correctly and consistently. Studies on serodiscordant couples (only one of whom is HIV-positive) have shown that, with regular sexual intercourse over a period of two years, partners who consistently use condoms have a near-zero risk of HIV infection.

A man should always use a condom during sexual intercourse, each time, from start to finish, and a woman should make sure that her partner uses one. A woman can also protect herself from sexually transmitted infections by using a female condom – essentially, a vaginal pouch – which is now commercially available in some countries.

It is essential to avoid injecting drugs for non-medical purposes, and particularly to avoid any type of needle-sharing to reduce the risk of acquiring hepatitis, HIV, syphilis and other infections from contaminated needles and blood.

Medical injections using unsterilized equipment are also a possible source of infection. If an injection is essential, the traveller should try to ensure that the needles and syringes come from a sterile package or have been sterilized properly by steam or boiling water for 20 minutes.

Patients under medical care who require frequent injections, e.g. diabetics, should carry sufficient sterile needles and syringes for the duration of their trip and a doctor's authorization for their use.

Unsterile dental and surgical instruments, needles used in acupuncture and tattooing, ear-piercing devices, and other skin-piercing instruments can likewise transmit infection and should be avoided.

Treatment

Travellers with signs or symptoms of a sexually transmitted disease should cease all sexual activity and seek medical care immediately. The absence of symptoms does not guarantee absence of infection, and travellers exposed to unprotected sex should be tested for infection on returning home. HIV testing should always be voluntary and with counselling.

The sexually transmitted infections caused by bacteria, e.g. chancroid, chlamydia, gonorrhoea and syphilis, can be treated successfully. However, throughout the world, many of these bacteria are showing increased resistance to penicillin and other antimicrobials.

Treatment for sexually transmitted viral infections, e.g. hepatitis B, genital herpes and genital warts, is unsatisfactory because of the lack of specific medication, and cure is difficult to achieve. The same is true of HIV infection, which in its late stage causes AIDS and is thought to be invariably fatal. Antiretroviral drugs cannot completely eradicate HIV infection; treatment is expensive and complex and most countries have only a few centres that are able to provide it.

INFLUENZA

Cause	Influenza viruses of types A, B and C; type A occurs in two principal subtypes (H1N1 and H3N2). Type A viruses cause most of the widespread influenza epidemics; type B viruses generally cause regional outbreaks, and type C cause common colds and bronchitis.
	Influenza viruses evolve rapidly, changing their antigenic characteristics, so that vaccines need to be modified each year to be effective against currently circulating influenza strains.
	Other subtypes of influenza A viruses occur in animals and all 16 HA and 9 NA subtypes occur in birds; inter-species transmission (1918 pandemic) and viral reassortment (1957, 1968 pandemics) may give rise to new subtypes able to infect humans.
Transmission	Respiratory transmission occurs by droplets disseminated by unprotected coughs and sneezes. Short-distance airborne transmission of influenza viruses may occur, particularly in crowded enclosed spaces. Hand contamination and direct inoculation of virus is another potential route of spread.
Nature of the disease	An acute respiratory infection of varying severity, ranging from asymptomatic infection to fatal disease. Classic influenza symptoms include fever with rapid onset, sore throat, cough and chills, often accompanied by headache, coryza, myalgia and prostration. Influenza may be complicated by viral or more often bacterial pneumonia. Illness tends to be most severe in the elderly and in infants and young children. Death resulting from seasonal influenza occurs mainly in the elderly and in individuals with pre-existing chronic diseases.
Geographical distribution	Worldwide. In temperate regions, influenza is a seasonal disease occurring typically in winter months: it affects the northern hemisphere from November to April and the southern hemisphere from April to September. In tropical areas there is no clear seasonal pattern, and influenza may occur at any time of the year. Activity may occur year-round in the tropics.
Risk for travellers	Travellers, like local residents, are at risk in any country during the influenza season. Travellers visiting countries in the opposite hemisphere during the influenza season are at special risk, particularly if they have not built up some degree of immunity through regular vaccination. The elderly, people with pre-existing chronic diseases and young children are most susceptible to complications.

Prophylaxis	Vaccination before the start of the influenza season. However, vaccine for visitors to the opposite hemisphere may not be obtainable before arrival at the travel destination (see Chapter 6).
	For travellers in the highest risk groups for severe influenza who have not been or cannot be vaccinated, the prophylactic use of antiviral drugs such as zanamivir or oseltamivir is indicated in countries where they are available. Amantadine and rimantadine may also be considered when the circulating strains are known to be susceptible. However, the latter drugs are not active against influenza B, and high frequencies of resistance in H3N2 and less often H1N1 viruses make then unreliable for prevention currently.
Precautions	Whenever possible, avoid crowded enclosed spaces and close contact with people suffering from acute respiratory infections. Hand-washing after direct contact with ill persons or their environment may reduce the risk of illness. Ill persons should be encouraged to practice cough etiquette (maintain distance, cover coughs and sneezes with disposable tissues or clothing, wash hands).

JAPANESE ENCEPHALITIS

Cause	Japanese encephalitis (JE) virus, which is a flavivirus.
Transmission	The virus is transmitted by various mosquitoes of the genus *Culex*. It infects pigs and various wild birds as well as humans. Mosquitoes become infective after feeding on viraemic pigs or birds.
Nature of the disease	Most infections are asymptomatic. In symptomatic cases, severity varies; mild infections are characterized by febrile headache or aseptic meningitis. Severe cases have a rapid onset and progression, with headache, high fever and meningeal signs. Permanent neurological sequelae are common among survivors. Approximately 50% of severe clinical cases have a fatal outcome.
Geographical distribution	JE occurs in a number of countries in Asia (see map) and occasionally in northern Queensland, Australia.
Risk for travellers	Low for most travellers. Visitors to rural and agricultural areas in endemic countries may be at risk, particularly during epidemics of JE.
Prophylaxis	Vaccination, if justified by likelihood of exposure (see Chapter 6).
Precautions	Avoid mosquito bites (see Chapter 3).

LEGIONELLOSIS

Cause	Various species of *Legionella* bacteria, frequently *Legionella pneumophila*, serogroup I.
Transmission	Infection results from inhalation of contaminated water sprays or mists. The bacteria live in water and colonize hot-water systems at temperatures of 20–50 °C (optimal 35–46 °C). They contaminate air-conditioning cooling towers, hot-water systems, humidifiers, whirlpool spas and other water-containing devices. There is no direct person-to-person transmission.

Nature of the disease	Legionellosis occurs in two distinct clinical forms:
	■ Legionnaires' disease is an acute bacterial pneumonia with rapid onset of anorexia, malaise, myalgia, headache and rapidly rising fever, progressing to pneumonia, which may lead to respiratory failure and death.
	■ Pontiac fever is an influenza-like illness with spontaneous recovery after 2–5 days.
	Susceptibility to legionellosis increases with age, especially among smokers and people with pre-existing chronic lung disease or other immunocompromising conditions.
Geographical distribution	Worldwide.
Risk for travellers	Generally low. Outbreaks occasionally occur through dissemination of infection by contaminated water or air-conditioning systems in hotels and other facilities used by visitors.
Prophylaxis	None. Prevention of infection depends on regular cleaning and disinfection of possible sources.
Precautions	None.

LEISHMANIASIS (INCLUDING ESPUNDIA OR ORIENTAL SORE, AND KALA-AZAR)

Cause	Several species of the protozoan parasite *Leishmania*.
Transmission	Infection is transmitted by the bite of female phlebotomine sandflies. Dogs, rodents and other mammals are reservoir hosts for leishmaniasis. Sandflies acquire the parasites by biting infected humans or animals. Transmission from person to person by injected blood or contaminated syringes and needles is also possible.
Nature of the disease	Leishmaniasis occurs in two main forms:
	■ Cutaneous and mucosal leishmaniasis (espundia) causes skin sores and chronic ulcers of the mucosae. Cutaneous leishmaniasis is a chronic, progressive, disabling and often mutilating disease.
	■ Visceral leishmaniasis (kala-azar) affects the bone marrow, liver, spleen, lymph nodes and other internal organs. It is usually fatal if untreated.
Geographical distribution	Many countries in tropical and subtropical regions, including Africa, parts of central and south America, Asia, southern Europe and the eastern Mediterranean. Over 90% of all cases of visceral leishmaniasis occur in Bangladesh, Brazil, India, Nepal and Sudan. More than 90% of all cases of cutaneous leishmaniasis occur in Afghanistan, Algeria, Brazil, the Islamic Republic of Iran, Saudi Arabia and the Syrian Arab Republic.
Risk for travellers	Visitors to rural and forested areas in endemic countries are at risk.
Prophylaxis	None.
Precautions	Avoid sandfly bites, particularly after sunset, by using repellents and insecticide-impregnated bednets. The bite leaves a non-swollen red ring, which can alert the traveller to its origin.

69

LEPTOSPIROSIS (INCLUDING WEIL DISEASE)

Cause	Various spirochaetes of the genus *Leptospira*.
Transmission	Infection occurs through contact between the skin (particularly skin abrasions) or mucous membranes and water, wet soil or vegetation contaminated by the urine of infected animals, notably rats. Occasionally infection may result from direct contact with urine or tissues of infected animals, or from consumption of food contaminated by the urine of infected rats.
Nature of the disease	Leptospiral infections take many different clinical forms, usually with sudden onset of fever, headache, myalgia, chills, conjunctival suffusion and skin rash. The disease may progress to meningitis, haemolytic anaemia, jaundice, haemorrhagic manifestations and other complications, including hepatorenal failure.
Geographical distribution	Worldwide. Most common in tropical countries.
Risk for travellers	Low for most travellers. There is occupational risk for farmers engaged in paddy rice and sugar cane production. Visitors to rural areas and in contact with water in canals, lakes and rivers may be exposed to infection. There is increased risk after recent floods. The risk may be greater for those who practise canoeing, kayaking or other activities in water.
Prophylaxis	None. Vaccine against local strains is available for workers where the disease is an occupational hazard but is not commercially available in most countries.
Precautions	Avoid swimming or wading in potentially contaminated waters including canals, ponds, rivers, streams and swamps. Avoid all direct or indirect contact with rodents.

LISTERIOSIS

Cause	The bacterium *Listeria monocytogenes*.
Transmission	Listeriosis affects a variety of animals. Foodborne infection in humans occurs through the consumption of contaminated foods, particularly unpasteurized milk, soft cheeses, vegetables and prepared meat products such as pâté. Listeriosis multiplies readily in refrigerated foods that have been contaminated, unlike most foodborne pathogens. Transmission can also occur from mother to fetus or from mother to child during birth.
Nature of the disease	Listeriosis causes meningoencephalitis and/or septicaemia in adults and newborn infants. In pregnant women, it causes fever and abortion. Newborn infants, pregnant women, the elderly and immunocompromised individuals are particularly susceptible to listeriosis. In others, the disease may be limited to a mild acute febrile episode. In pregnant women, transmission of infection to the fetus may lead to stillbirth, septicaemia at birth or neonatal meningitis.
Geographical distribution	Worldwide, with sporadic incidence.
Risk for travellers	Generally low. Risk is increased by consumption of unpasteurized milk and milk products and prepared meat products.

Prophylaxis	None.
Precautions	Avoid consumption of unpasteurized milk and milk products. Pregnant women and immunocompromised individuals should take stringent precautions to avoid infection by listeriosis and other foodborne pathogens (see Chapter 3).

LYME BORRELIOSIS (LYME DISEASE)

Cause	The spirochaete *Borrelia burgdorferi*, of which there are several different serotypes.
Transmission	Infection occurs through the bite of infected ticks, both adults and nymphs, of the genus *Ixodes*. Most human infections result from bites by nymphs. Many species of mammals can be infected, and deer act as an important reservoir.
Nature of the disease	The disease usually has its onset in summer. Early skin lesions have an expanding ring form, often with a central clear zone. Fever, chills, myalgia and headache are common. Meningeal involvement may follow. Central nervous system and other complications may occur weeks or months after the onset of illness. Arthritis may develop up to 2 years after onset.
Geographical distribution	There are endemic foci of Lyme borreliosis in forested areas of Asia, northwestern, central and eastern Europe, and the USA.
Risk for travellers	Generally low. Visitors to rural areas in endemic regions, particularly campers and hikers, are at risk.
Prophylaxis	None.
Precautions	Avoid tick-infested areas and exposure to ticks (see Chapter 3). If a bite occurs, remove the tick as soon as possible.

MALARIA

See Chapter 7 and map.

MENINGOCOCCAL DISEASE

Cause	The bacterium *Neisseria meningitidis*, of which 12 serogroups are known. Most cases of meningococcal disease are caused by serogroups A, B and C; less commonly, infection is caused by serogroups Y and W-135. Epidemics in Africa are usually caused by *N. meningitidis* type A.
Transmission	Transmission occurs by direct person-to-person contact, including aerosol transmission and respiratory droplets from the nose and pharynx of infected persons, patients or asymptomatic carriers. There is no animal reservoir or insect vector.
Nature of the disease	Most infections do not cause clinical disease. Many infected people become asymptomatic carriers of the bacteria and serve as a reservoir and source of infection for others. In general, susceptibility to meningococcal disease decreases with age, although there is a small increase in risk in adolescents

and young adults. Meningococcal meningitis has a sudden onset of intense headache, fever, nausea, vomiting, photophobia and stiff neck, plus various neurological signs. The disease is fatal in 5–10% of cases even with prompt antimicrobial treatment in good health care facilities; among individuals who survive, up to 20% have permanent neurological sequelae. Meningococcal septicaemia, in which there is rapid dissemination of bacteria in the bloodstream, is a less common form of meningococcal disease, characterized by circulatory collapse, haemorrhagic skin rash and high fatality rate.

Geographical distribution	Sporadic cases are found worldwide. In temperate zones, most cases occur in the winter months. Localized outbreaks occur in enclosed crowded spaces (e.g. dormitories, military barracks). In sub-Saharan Africa, in a zone stretching across the continent from Senegal to Ethiopia (the African "meningitis belt"), large outbreaks and epidemics take place during the dry season (November–June). Meningococcal serogroups A, B and C are responsible for the vast majority of cases worldwide. Serogroup A is the cause of most major epidemics. In most parts of the world, serogroups Y and W-135 are relatively uncommon causes of meningococcal infection. However, recent reports of endemic occurrence of group Y meningococcal disease in the United States, and outbreaks caused by serogroup W-135 strains in Saudi Arabia and sub-Saharan Africa, particularly Burkina Faso, suggest that these serogroups may be gaining in importance.
Risk for travellers	Generally low. However, the risk is considerable if travellers are in crowded conditions or take part in large population movements such as pilgrimages in the Sahel meningitis belt. Localized outbreaks occasionally occur among travellers (usually young adults) in camps or dormitories. See also Chapter 6 for specific risks for travellers.
Prophylaxis	Vaccination is available for *N. meningitidis* types A, C, Y and W-135 (see Chapter 6). Protection by vaccines is group-specific, and appropriate vaccines need to be administered to protect against the most prevalent serogroup at the destination country of the traveller.
Precautions	Avoid overcrowding in confined spaces. Following close contact with a person suffering from meningococcal disease, medical advice should be sought regarding chemoprophylaxis.

PLAGUE

Cause	The plague bacillus, *Yersinia pestis*.
Transmission	Plague is a zoonotic disease affecting rodents and transmitted by fleas from rodents to other animals and to humans. Direct person-to-person transmission does not occur except in the case of pneumonic plague, when respiratory droplets may transfer the infection from the patient to others in close contact.
Nature of the disease	Plague occurs in three main clinical forms: ■ Bubonic plague is the form that usually results from the bite of infected fleas. Lymphadenitis develops in the drainage lymph nodes, with the regional lymph nodes most commonly affected. Swelling, pain and suppuration of the lymph nodes produces the characteristic plague buboes.

■ Septicaemic plague may develop from bubonic plague or occur in the absence of lymphadenitis. Dissemination of the infection in the bloodstream results in meningitis, endotoxic shock and disseminated intravascular coagulation.

■ Pneumonic plague may result from secondary infection of the lungs following dissemination of plague bacilli from other body sites. It produces severe pneumonia. Direct infection of others may result from transfer of infection by respiratory droplets, causing primary pulmonary plague in the recipients.

Without prompt and effective treatment, 50–60% of cases of bubonic plague are fatal, while untreated septicaemic and pneumonic plague are invariably fatal.

Geographical distribution	There are natural foci of plague infection of rodents in many parts of the world. Wild rodent plague is present in central, eastern and southern Africa, south America, the western part of north America and in large areas of Asia. In some areas, contact between wild and domestic rats is common, resulting in sporadic cases of human plague and occasional outbreaks.
Risk for travellers	Generally low. However, travellers in rural areas of plague-endemic regions may be at risk, particularly if camping or hunting or if contact with rodents takes place.
Prophylaxis	A vaccine effective against bubonic plague is available exclusively for persons with a high occupational exposure to plague; it is not commercially available in most countries.
Precautions	Avoid any contact with live or dead rodents.

RABIES

Cause	The rabies virus, a rhabdovirus of the genus *Lyssavirus*.
Transmission	Rabies is a zoonotic disease affecting a wide range of domestic and wild animals, including bats. Infection of humans usually occurs through the bite of an infected animal as the virus is present in the saliva. Any other contact with a rabies-susceptible species such as a penetrating scratch with bleeding and licking of broken skin and mucosa in an area where rabies is present should be treated with caution. In developing countries transmission is usually through dog bites. Person-to-person transmission has not been laboratory-confirmed.
Nature of the disease	An acute viral encephalomyelitis, which is almost invariably fatal. The initial signs include a sense of apprehension, headache, fever, malaise and sensory changes around the site of the animal bite. Excitability, hallucinations and aerophobia are common, followed in some cases by fear of water (hydrophobia) due to spasms of the swallowing muscles, progressing to delirium, convulsions and death a few days after onset. A less common form, paralytic rabies, is characterized by loss of sensation, weakness, pain and paralysis.
Geographical distribution	Rabies is present in animals in many countries worldwide (see map). Most of the estimated 55 000 rabies deaths per year in Africa and Asia alone occur in developing countries and follow a dog bite.

Risk for travellers	In rabies-endemic areas, travellers may be at risk if there is a mild or severe exposure to a rabies-susceptible animal species (domestic, particularly dogs and cats, or wild, including bats).
Prophylaxis	Vaccination for travellers with a foreseeable significant risk of exposure to rabies or travelling to a hyperendemic area where modern rabies vaccine may not be available (see Chapter 6).
Precautions	Avoid contact with wild animals and stray domestic animals, particularly dogs and cats, in rabies-endemic areas. If bitten by an animal that is potentially infected with rabies, or after other suspect contact as defined above, immediately clean the wound thoroughly with disinfectant or with soap or detergent and water. Medical assistance should be sought immediately.

The vaccination status of the animal involved should not be a criterion for withholding post-exposure prophylaxis unless the vaccination has been thoroughly documented and vaccine of known potency has been used. In the case of domestic animals, the suspect animal should be kept under observation for a period of 10 days. After 10 days, if the animal under observation is healthy, post-exposure prophylaxis can be stopped. |

SARS (SEVERE ACUTE RESPIRATORY SYNDROME)

Cause	SARS coronavirus (SARS-CoV) – virus identified in 2003. SARS-CoV is thought to be an animal virus from an as–yet uncertain–animal reservoir, which first infected humans in the Guangdong province of southern China in 2002.
Transmission	An epidemic of SARS affected 26 countries and resulted in over 8000 cases in 2003. Since then, a small number of cases have occurred as a result of laboratory accidents or, possibly, through animal-to-human transmission (Guangdong, China).

Transmission of SARS-CoV was primarily from person-to-person. It occurs mainly during the second week of illness, which corresponds to the peak of virus excretion in respiratory secretions and stool, and when cases with severe disease start to deteriorate clinically. |
| Nature of the disease | Symptoms were flu-like and included fever, malaise, muscle aches and pains (myalgia), headache, diarrhoea, and shivering (rigors). No individual symptom or cluster of symptoms has proved to be specific for a diagnosis of SARS. Although fever was the most frequently reported symptom, it was sometimes absent on initial measurement.

Cough (initially dry), shortness of breath, and diarrhoea presented in the first and/or second week of illness. Severe cases often developed rapidly, progressing to respiratory distress and requiring intensive care. |
| Geographical distribution | The distribution is based on the 2002–2003 epidemic. The disease appeared in November 2002 in the Guangdong province of southern China. This area is considered as a potential zone of re-emergence of SARS-CoV.

Other countries/areas in which chains of human-to-human transmission occurred after early importation of cases were Hong Kong Special Administrative Region and Taiwan in China, Toronto in Canada, Singapore, and Hanoi in Viet Nam. In other countries, imported cases did not lead to local outbreaks. |

Risk for travellers	Currently, no areas of the world are reporting transmission of SARS. Since the end of the global epidemic in July 2003, SARS has reappeared four times – three times from laboratory accidents (Singapore, Taiwan, China), and once in southern China where the source of infection remains undetermined although there is circumstantial evidence of animal-to-human transmission.
	Should SARS re-emerge in epidemic form, WHO will provide guidance on the risk of travel to affected areas. Travellers should stay informed about current travel recommendations. However, even during the height of the 2003 epidemic, the overall risk of SARS-CoV transmission to travellers was low.
Prophylaxis	None.
Precautions	Follow any travel recommendations and health advice issued by WHO.

SCHISTOSOMIASIS (BILHARZIASIS)

Cause	Several species of parasitic blood flukes (trematodes), of which the most important are *Schistosoma mansoni*, *S. japonicum* and *S. haematobium*.
Transmission	Infection occurs in fresh water containing larval forms (cercariae) of schistosomes, which develop in snails. The free-swimming larvae penetrate the skin of individuals swimming or wading in water. Snails become infected as a result of excretion of eggs in human urine or faeces.
Nature of the disease	Chronic conditions in which adult flukes live for many years in the veins (mesenteric or vesical) of the host where they produce eggs, which cause damage to the organs in which they are deposited. The symptoms depend on the main target organs affected by the different species, with *S. mansoni* and *S. japonicum* causing hepatic and intestinal signs and *S. haematobium* causing urinary dysfunction. The larvae of some schistosomes of birds and other animals may penetrate human skin and cause a self-limiting dermatitis, "swimmers itch". These larvae are unable to develop in humans.
Geographical distribution	*S. mansoni* occurs in many countries of sub-Saharan Africa, in the Arabian peninsula, and in Brazil, Suriname and Venezuela. *S. japonicum* is found in China, in parts of Indonesia, and in the Philippines (but no longer in Japan). *S. haematobium* is present in sub-Saharan Africa and in eastern Mediterranean areas. *S. mekongi* is found along the Mekong River in northern Cambodia and in the south of the Lao People's Democratic Republic.
Risk for travellers	In endemic areas, travellers are at risk while swimming or wading in fresh water.
Prophylaxis	None.
Precautions	Avoid direct contact (swimming or wading) with potentially contaminated fresh water in endemic areas. In case of accidental exposure, dry the skin vigorously to reduce penetration by cercariae. Avoid drinking, washing, or washing clothing in water that may contain cercariae. Water can be treated to remove or inactivate cercariae by paper filtering or use of iodine or chlorine.

TICK-BORNE ENCEPHALITIS (SPRING–SUMMER ENCEPHALITIS)

Cause	The tick-borne encephalitis (TBE) virus, which is a flavivirus. Other closely related viruses cause similar diseases.
Transmission	Infection is transmitted by the bite of infected ticks. There is no direct person-to-person transmission. Some related viruses, also tick-borne, infect animals such as birds, deer (louping-ill), rodents and sheep.
Nature of the disease	Infection may induce an influenza-like illness, with a second phase of fever occurring in 10% of cases. Encephalitis develops during the second phase and may result in paralysis, permanent sequelae or death. Severity of illness increases with age.
Geographical distribution	Present in large parts of Europe, particularly Austria, the Baltic states (Estonia, Latvia, Lithuania), the Czech Republic, Hungary and the Russian Federation. The disease is seasonal, occurring mainly during the summer months in rural and forest areas at altitudes up to 1000 metres.
Risk for travellers	In endemic areas during the summer months, travellers are at risk when hiking or camping in rural or forest areas.
Prophylaxis	A vaccine against TBE is available (see Chapter 6).
Precautions	Avoid bites by ticks by wearing long trousers and closed footwear when hiking or camping in endemic areas. If a bite occurs, the tick should be removed as soon as possible.

TRYPANOSOMIASIS

1. African trypanosomiasis (sleeping sickness)

Cause	Protozoan parasites *Trypanosoma brucei gambiense* and *T. b. rhodesiense*.
Transmission	Infection occurs through the bite of infected tsetse flies. Humans are the main reservoir host for *T. b. gambiense*. Domestic cattle and wild animals, including antelopes, are the main animal reservoir of *T. b. rhodesiense*.
Nature of the disease	*T. b. gambiense* causes a chronic illness with onset of symptoms after a prolonged incubation period of weeks or months. *T. b. rhodesiense* causes a more acute illness, with onset a few days or weeks after the infected bite; often, there is a striking inoculation chancre. Initial clinical signs include severe headache, insomnia, enlarged lymph nodes, anaemia and rash. In the late stage of the disease, there is progressive loss of weight and involvement of the central nervous system. Without treatment, the disease is invariably fatal.
Geographical distribution	*T. b. gambiense* is present in foci in the tropical countries of western and central Africa. *T. b. rhodesiense* occurs in east Africa, extending south as far as Botswana.
Risk for travellers	Travellers are at risk in endemic regions if they visit rural areas for hunting, fishing, safari trips, sailing or other activities in endemic areas.
Prophylaxis	None.

Precautions	Travellers should be aware of the risk in endemic areas and as far as possible avoid any contact with tsetse flies. However, bites are difficult to avoid because tsetse flies can bite through clothing. Travellers should be warned that tsetse flies bite during the day and are not repelled by available insect-repellent products. The bite is painful, which helps to identify its origin, and travellers should seek medical attention promptly if symptoms develop subsequently.

2. American trypanosomiasis (Chagas disease)

Cause	Protozoan parasite *Trypanosoma cruzi*.
Transmission	Infection is transmitted by blood-sucking triatomine bugs ("kissing bugs"). Oral transmission by ingestion of unprocessed freshly squeezed sugar cane in areas where the vector is present has also been reported. During feeding, infected bugs excrete trypanosomes, which can then contaminate the conjunctiva, mucous membranes, abrasions and skin wounds including the bite wound. Transmission also occurs by blood transfusion when blood has been obtained from an infected donor. Congenital infection is possible, due to parasites crossing the placenta during pregnancy. *T. cruzi* infects many species of wild and domestic animals as well as humans.
Nature of the disease	In adults, *T. cruzi* causes a chronic illness with progressive myocardial damage leading to cardiac arrhythmias and cardiac dilatation, and gastrointestinal involvement leading to mega-oesophagus and megacolon. *T. cruzi* causes acute illness in children, which is followed by chronic manifestations later in life.
Geographical distribution	American trypanosomiasis occurs in Mexico and in central and south America (as far south as central Argentina and Chile). The vector is found mainly in rural areas where it lives in the walls of poorly-constructed housing.
Risk for travellers	In endemic areas, travellers are at risk when trekking, camping or using poor-quality housing.
Precautions	Avoid exposure to blood-sucking bugs. Residual insecticides can be used to treat housing. Exposure can be reduced by the use of bednets in houses and camps.

TUBERCULOSIS

Cause	*Mycobacterium tuberculosis*, the tubercle bacillus. Humans can also become infected by bovine tuberculosis, caused by *M. bovis*.
Transmission	Infection is usually by direct airborne transmission from person to person.
Nature of the disease	Exposure to *M. tuberculosis* may lead to infection, but most infections do not lead to disease. The risk of developing disease following infection is generally 5–10% during the lifetime, but may be increased by various factors, notably immunosuppression (e.g. advanced HIV infection).
	Multidrug resistance refers to strains of *M. tuberculosis* that are resistant to at least isoniazid and rifampicin (MDR-TB). The resistant strains do not differ from other strains in infectiousness, likelihood of causing disease, or general clinical effects; however, if they do cause disease, treatment is more

	difficult and the risk of death will be higher. Extensively drug-resistant TB (XDR-TB) is TB that is resistant to at least isoniazid and rifampin and to any fluoroquinolone and to at least one of the injectable second-line anti-TB drugs capreomycin, kanamycin, amikacin.
Geographical distribution	Worldwide. The risk of infection differs between countries, as shown on the map of estimated TB incidence.
Risk for travellers	Low for most travellers. Long-term travellers (over 3 months) to a country with a higher incidence of tuberculosis than their own may have a risk of infection comparable to that for local residents. As well as the duration of the visit, living conditions are important in determining the risk of infection: high-risk settings include health facilities, shelters for the homeless, and prisons.
Prophylaxis	BCG vaccine is of limited use for travellers but may be advised for infants and young children in some situations (see Chapter 6).
Precautions	Travellers should avoid close contact with known tuberculosis patients. For travellers from low-incidence countries who may be exposed to infection in relatively high-incidence countries (e.g. health professionals, humanitarian relief workers, missionaries), a baseline tuberculin skin test is advisable in order to compare with retesting after return. If the skin reaction to tuberculin suggests recent infection, the traveller should receive, or be referred for, treatment for latent infection. Patients under treatment for tuberculosis should not travel until the treating physician has documented, by laboratory examination of sputum, that the patient is not infectious and therefore of no risk to others. The importance of completing the prescribed course of treatment should be stressed.

TYPHOID FEVER

Cause	*Salmonella typhi*, the typhoid bacillus, which infects only humans. Similar paratyphoid and enteric fevers are caused by other species of *Salmonella*, which infect domestic animals as well as humans.
Transmission	Infection is transmitted by consumption of contaminated food or water. Occasionally direct faecal–oral transmission may occur. Shellfish taken from sewage-polluted beds are an important source of infection. Infection occurs through eating fruit and vegetables fertilized by night soil and eaten raw, and milk and milk products that have been contaminated by those in contact with them. Flies may transfer infection to foods, resulting in contamination that may be sufficient to cause human infection. Pollution of water sources may produce epidemics of typhoid fever, when large numbers of people use the same source of drinking-water.
Nature of the disease	A systemic disease of varying severity. Severe cases are characterized by gradual onset of fever, headache, malaise, anorexia and insomnia. Constipation is more common than diarrhoea in adults and older children. Without treatment, the disease progresses with sustained fever, bradycardia, hepatosplenomegaly, abdominal symptoms and, in some cases, pneumonia. In white-skinned patients, pink spots (papules), which fade on pressure, appear on the skin of the trunk in up to 50% of cases. In the third week, untreated

	cases develop additional gastrointestinal and other complications, which may prove fatal. Around 2–5% of those who contract typhoid fever become chronic carriers, as bacteria persist in the biliary tract after symptoms have resolved.
Geographical distribution	Worldwide. The disease occurs most commonly in association with poor standards of hygiene in food preparation and handling and where sanitary disposal of sewage is lacking.
Risk for travellers	Generally low risk for travellers, except in parts of north and west Africa, in south Asia and in Peru. Elsewhere, travellers are usually at risk only when exposed to low standards of hygiene with respect to food handling, control of drinking-water quality, and sewage disposal.
Prophylaxis	Vaccination (see Chapter 6).
Precautions	Observe all precautions against exposure to foodborne and waterborne infections (see Chapter 3).

TYPHUS FEVER (EPIDEMIC LOUSE-BORNE TYPHUS)

Cause	*Rickettsia prowazekii*.
Transmission	The disease is transmitted by the human body louse, which becomes infected by feeding on the blood of patients with acute typhus fever. Infected lice excrete rickettsia onto the skin while feeding on a second host, who becomes infected by rubbing louse faecal matter or crushed lice into the bite wound. There is no animal reservoir.
Nature of the disease	The onset is variable but often sudden, with headache, chills, high fever, prostration, coughing and severe muscular pain. After 5–6 days, a macular skin eruption (dark spots) develops first on the upper trunk and spreads to the rest of the body but usually not to the face, palms of the hands or soles of the feet. The case-fatality rate is up to 40% in the absence of specific treatment. Louse-borne typhus fever is the only rickettsial disease that can cause explosive epidemics.
Geographical distribution	Typhus fever occurs in colder (i.e. mountainous) regions of central and east Africa, central and south America, and Asia. In recent years, most outbreaks have taken place in Burundi, Ethiopia and Rwanda. Typhus fever occurs in conditions of overcrowding and poor hygiene, such as prisons and refugee camps.
Risk for travellers	Very low for most travellers. Humanitarian relief workers may be exposed in refugee camps and other settings characterized by crowding and poor hygiene.
Prophylaxis	None.
Precautions	Cleanliness is important in preventing infestation by body lice. Insecticidal powders are available for body-louse control and treatment of clothing for those at high risk of exposure.

YELLOW FEVER

Cause	The yellow fever virus, an arbovirus of the *Flavivirus* genus.
Transmission	Yellow fever in urban and some rural areas is transmitted by the bite of infective *Aedes aegypti* mosquitoes and by other mosquitoes in the forests of south America. The mosquitoes bite during daylight hours. Transmission occurs at altitudes up to 2500 metres. Yellow fever virus infects humans and monkeys.
	In jungle and forest areas, monkeys are the main reservoir of infection, with transmission from monkey to monkey carried out by mosquitoes. The infective mosquitoes may bite humans who enter the forest area, usually causing sporadic cases or small outbreaks.
	In urban areas, monkeys are not involved and infection is transmitted among humans by mosquitoes. Introduction of infection into densely populated urban areas can lead to large epidemics of yellow fever.
	In Africa, an intermediate pattern of transmission is common in humid savannah regions. Mosquitoes infect both monkeys and humans, causing localized outbreaks.
Nature of the disease	Although some infections are asymptomatic, most lead to an acute illness characterized by two phases. Initially, there is fever, muscular pain, headache, chills, anorexia, nausea and/or vomiting, often with bradycardia. About 15% of patients progress to a second phase after a few days, with resurgence of fever, development of jaundice, abdominal pain, vomiting and haemorrhagic manifestations; half of these patients die 10–14 days after onset of illness.
Geographical distribution	The yellow fever virus is endemic in some tropical areas of Africa and central and south America (see map). The number of epidemics has increased since the early 1980s. Other countries are considered to be at risk of introduction of yellow fever due to the presence of the vector and suitable primate hosts (including Asia, where yellow fever has never been reported).
Risk for travellers	Travellers are at risk in all areas where yellow fever is endemic. The risk is greatest for visitors who enter forest and jungle areas.
Prophylaxis	Vaccination (see Chapter 6). In some countries, yellow fever vaccination is mandatory for visitors (see Country list).
Precautions	Avoid mosquito bites during the day as well as at night (see Chapter 3).

Further reading

Disease outbreak news: http://www.who.int/csr/don/en

Heymann D, ed. *Control of communicable diseases manual*, 18th ed. Washington, DC, American Public Health Association, 2005.

Weekly epidemiological record: http://www.who.int/wer/

WHO information on infectious diseases: http://www.who.int/csr/disease/en

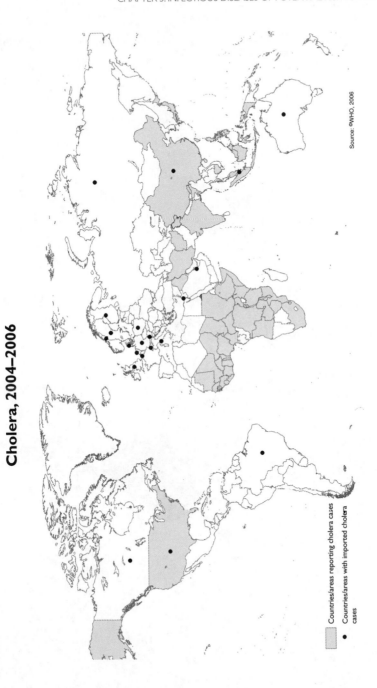

Cholera, 2004–2006

Source: ©WHO, 2006

Countries/areas reporting cholera cases

● Countries/areas with imported cholera cases

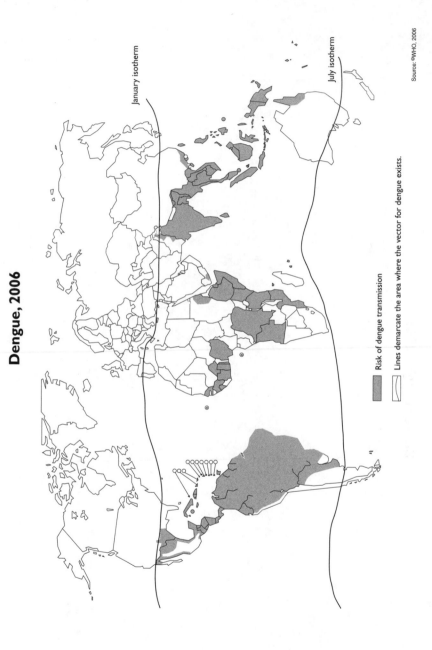

Dengue, 2006

January isotherm

July isotherm

Source: ©WHO, 2006

■ Risk of dengue transmission

Lines demarcate the area where the vector for dengue exists.

Hepatitis A, 2003

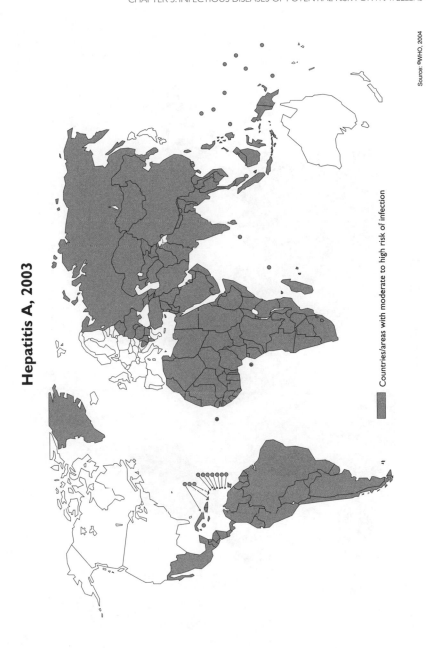

Source: ©WHO, 2004

Countries/areas with moderate to high risk of infection

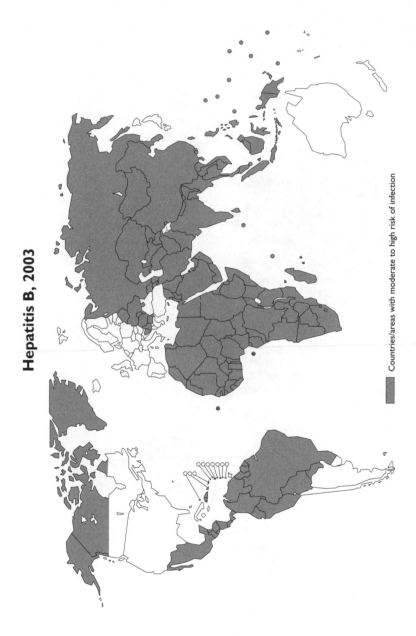

Hepatitis B, 2003

Source: ©WHO, 2004

Countries/areas with moderate to high risk of infection

Hepatitis C, 2003

Source: ©WHO, 2004

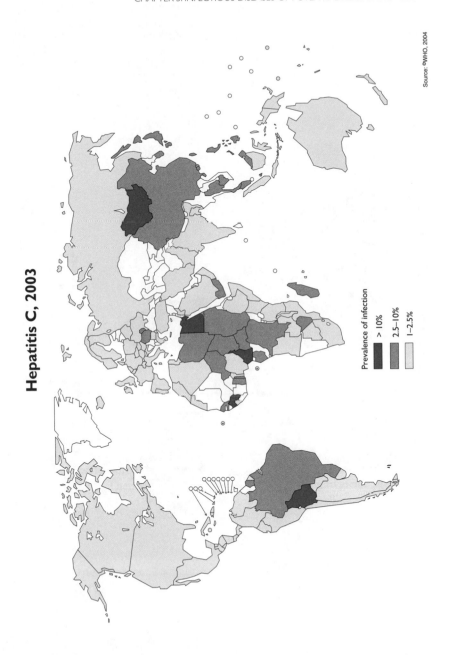

Prevalence of infection

> 10%

2.5–10%

1–2.5%

HIV infection, 2005

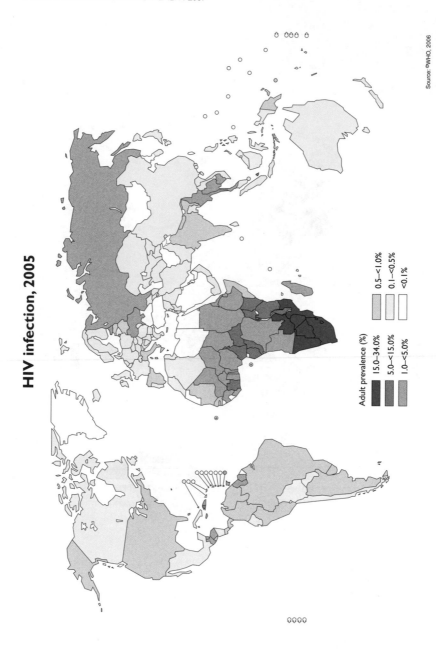

Source: ©WHO, 2006

Adult prevalence (%)

- 15.0–34.0%
- 5.0–<15.0%
- 1.0–<5.0%
- 0.5–<1.0%
- 0.1–<0.5%
- <0.1%

Japanese encephalitis, 2005

All-year transmission

Seasonal transmission

Source: ©WHO, 2004

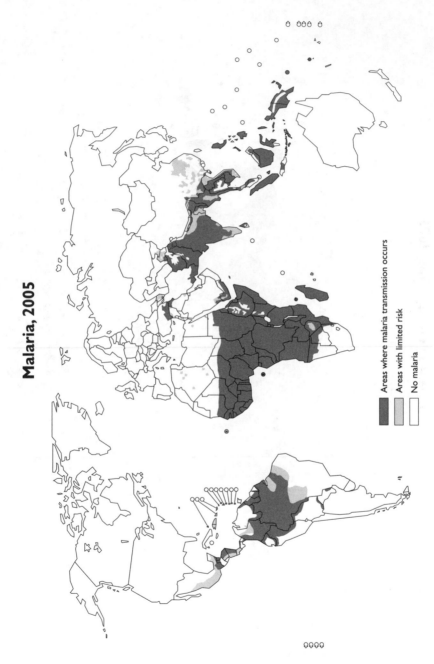

Malaria, 2005

Areas where malaria transmission occurs

Areas with limited risk

No malaria

Poliomyelitis, 2006

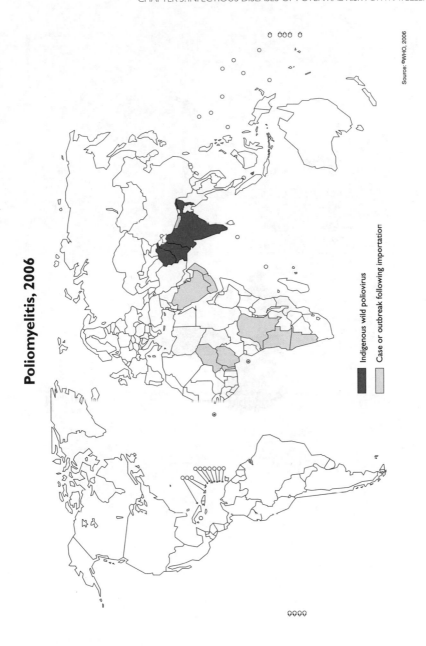

Source: ©WHO, 2006

Indigenous wild poliovirus

Case or outbreak following importation

Rabies, 2005

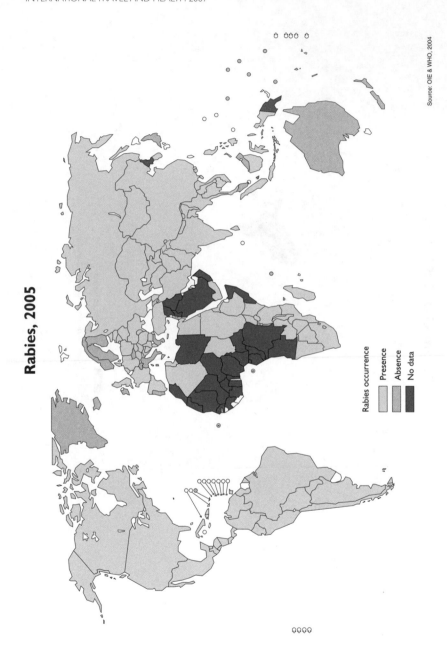

Rabies occurrence

Presence
Absence
No data

Source: OIE & WHO, 2004

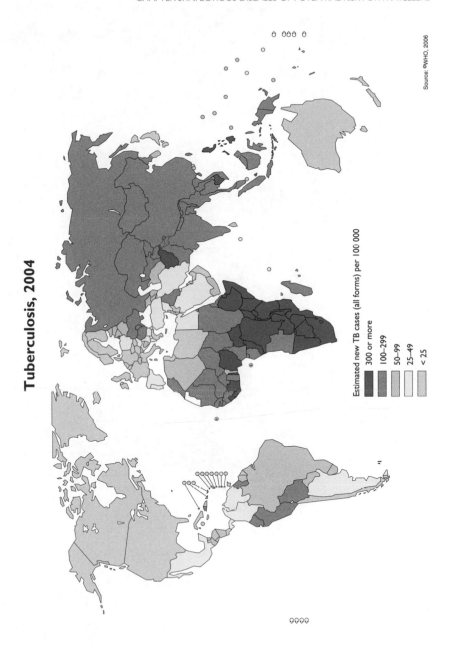

Tuberculosis, 2004

Source: ©WHO, 2006

Estimated new TB cases (all forms) per 100 000

300 or more
100–299
50–99
25–49
< 25

Yellow fever, 2005

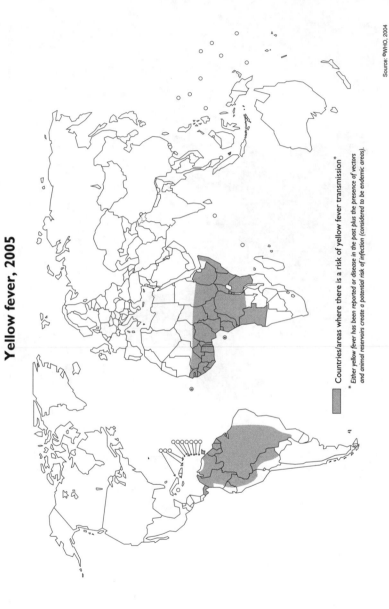

Source: ©WHO, 2004

- Countries/areas where there is a risk of yellow fever transmission*

* Either yellow fever has been reported or disease in the past plus the presence of vectors and animal reservoirs create a potential risk of infection (considered to be endemic areas).

CHAPTER 6

Vaccine-preventable diseases and vaccines

General considerations

Vaccination is the administration of a vaccine to stimulate a protective immune response that will prevent disease in the vaccinated person if contact with the corresponding infectious agent occurs subsequently. Thus vaccination, if successful, results in immunization: the vaccinated person has been rendered immune to disease caused by the infectious pathogen. In practice, the terms "vaccination" and "immunization" are often used interchangeably.

Disease prevention

Vaccination is a highly effective method of preventing certain infectious diseases. For the individual, and for society in terms of public health, prevention is better and more cost-effective than cure. Vaccines are generally very safe and serious adverse reactions are uncommon. Routine immunization programmes protect most of the world's children from a number of infectious diseases that previously claimed millions of lives each year. For travellers, vaccination offers the possibility of avoiding a number of dangerous diseases that may be encountered abroad. However, vaccines have not yet been developed against several of the most life-threatening infections, including malaria and HIV/AIDS.

Vaccination and other precautions

Despite their success in preventing disease, vaccines do not fully protect 100% of the recipients. The vaccinated traveller should not assume that there is no risk of contracting the disease(s) against which he/she has been vaccinated. All additional precautions against infection (see Chapter 5) should be followed carefully, regardless of any vaccines or other medication that have been administered. These same precautions are important in reducing the risk of acquiring diseases for which no vaccines exist and that represent health problems commonly faced by international travellers. It is also important to remember that immunization is not a substitute for avoiding potentially contaminated food and water

Planning before travel

Before departure, travellers should be advised about the risk of disease in the country or countries they plan to visit and the steps to be taken to prevent illness. The risk to a traveller of acquiring a disease depends on the local prevalence of that disease and on several other factors such as: age, sex, immunization status and current state of health; travel itinerary, duration and style of travel (e.g. first class, adventure, hiking, relief work).

Based on the traveller's individual risk assessment, a health care professional can determine the need for immunizations and/or preventive medication (prophylaxis) and provide advice on precautions to avoid disease.

There is no single schedule for the administration of immunizing agents to all travellers. Each schedule must be personalized and tailored to the individual traveller's immunization history, the countries to be visited, the type and duration of travel, and the amount of time available before departure.

Travel is a good opportunity for the health care provider to review the immunization status of infants, children, adolescents and adults. Un-immunized or incompletely immunized travellers should be offered the routine vaccinations recommended in national immunization schedules, in addition to those needed for travel.

The protective effect of many vaccines takes some time to develop following vaccination. The immune response of the vaccinated individual will become fully effective within a period of time that varies with the vaccine, the number of doses required and whether the individual has previously been vaccinated against the same disease. For this reason, travellers are advised to consult a travel medicine practitioner or physician 4–8 weeks before departure in order to allow sufficient time for optimal immunization schedules to be completed. However, an imminent departure still provides the opportunity to provide both advice and possibly some immunizations.

Vaccine schedules and administration

The vaccines that may be recommended or considered for travellers are shown in Table 6.1. The schedule for administration of each vaccine is given, together with other information for each of the vaccine-preventable diseases. Time intervals for administration of vaccines requiring more than one dose are recommended; some slight variation can be made to accommodate the needs of travellers who may not be able to complete the schedule exactly as recommended. In general, it is acceptable to lengthen the time intervals between doses, but significant shortening of the intervals is not recommended.

The route of administration differs for individual vaccines and is critical for induction of the protective immune response. For injectable vaccines, the route of injection – subcutaneous, intramuscular or intradermal – determines the gauge and length of the needle to be used. Intramuscular injections should be given in the anterolateral aspect of the thigh for infants and children under 2 years of age, and in the deltoid muscle for older children and adults; injection into the buttock is not recommended.

Safe injections

The same high standard of injection safety should be applied to the administration of vaccines as to any other injection. A sterile needle and syringe should be used for each injection and disposed of safely.

WHO recommends the use of single-use ("auto-disable") syringes or disposable monodose preparations whenever possible. Syringes should not be recapped (to avoid needle-stick injuries) and should be disposed of in a way that is safe for the recipient, the provider and the community.

Multiple vaccines

Inactivated vaccines do not generally interfere with other inactivated or live vaccines and can be given simultaneously with, or at any time in relation to, other vaccines without prejudicing immune responses. Most live vaccines can be given simultaneously. However, if two injected live-virus vaccines are not administered on the same day, the two injections should be separated by an interval of at least 4 weeks. The Ty21a typhoid vaccine can be administered simultaneously with or at any interval before or after other live vaccines.

A number of combination vaccines are now available, providing protection against more than one disease, and new combinations are likely to become available in future years. For routine vaccination, the combined diphtheria/tetanus/pertussis (DTP) and measles/mumps/rubella (MMR) vaccines are in widespread use in children. Other examples of combination vaccines are hepatitis A+B and hepatitis A + typhoid, IPV+DTP, IPV+DTP+Hib, MMR+varicella, IPV+DTP+HepB+Hib.[1] In adults, the combined diphtheria–tetanus vaccine (with reduced diphtheria, Td) is generally used in preference to monovalent tetanus toxoid vaccine. Combina-

---

[1] DTP= diphtheria, tetanus, pertussis; IPV = inactivated poliomyelitis vaccine; Hib = *Haemophilus influenzae* type b [vaccine]; HepB = hepatitis B [vaccine]; MMR= measles, mumps, rubella

tion vaccines offer important advantages for travellers, by reducing the number of injections required and the amount of time involved, so aiding compliance. Combination vaccines are just as safe and effective as the individual single-disease vaccines.

Choice of vaccines for travel

Vaccines for travellers include: (1) those that are used routinely, particularly but not only in children; (2) others that may be advised before travel to disease-endemic countries; (3) those that, in some situations, are mandatory.

Most of the vaccines that are routinely administered in childhood require periodic booster doses throughout life to maintain an effective level of immunity. Adults in their country of residence often neglect to keep up the schedule of booster vaccinations, particularly if the risk of infection is low. Some older adults may never have been vaccinated at all. It is important to realize that diseases such as diphtheria and poliomyelitis, which no longer occur in most industrialized countries, may be present in those visited by travellers. Pre-travel precautions should include booster doses of routine vaccines if the regular schedule has not been followed, or a full course of primary immunization for people who have never been vaccinated.

Other vaccines will be advised on the basis of a travel risk assessment for the individual traveller (see also Chapter 1). In deciding which vaccines would be appropriate, the following factors are to be considered for each vaccine:

- risk of exposure to the disease
- age, health status, vaccination history
- reactions to previous vaccine doses, allergies
- risk of infecting others
- cost.

Mandatory vaccination, as authorized by the International Health Regulations, nowadays concerns only yellow fever. Yellow fever vaccination is carried out for two different reasons: (1) to protect the individual in areas where there is a risk of yellow fever infection; and (2) to protect vulnerable countries from importation of the yellow fever virus. Travellers should therefore be vaccinated if they visit a country where there is a risk of exposure to yellow fever. They must be vaccinated if they visit a country that requires yellow fever vaccination as a condition of entry; this condition applies to all travellers who arrive from (including airport transit) a yellow fever endemic country.

Vaccination against meningococcal disease is required by Saudi Arabia for pilgrims visiting Mecca annually (Hajj) or at any time (Umrah) and/or Medina.

Table 6.1 **Vaccines for travellers**

Category	Vaccine
1. Routine vaccination	Diphtheria, tetanus, and pertussis Hepatitis B *Haemophilus influenzae* type b Human papillomavirus[a] Influenza[b] Measles, mumps and rubella Pneumococcal disease Poliomyelitis Rotavirus[a] Tuberculosis (BCG)[c] Varicella
2. Selective use for travellers	Cholera Hepatitis A[d] Japanese encephalitis[d] Meningococcal disease[d] Rabies Tick-borne encephalitis Typhoid fever Yellow fever[d]
3. Mandatory vaccination	Yellow fever (see country list) Meningococcal disease and polio (required by Saudi Arabia for pilgrims; updates are available on http://www.who.int/wer)

[a] These vaccines are currently being introduced in some countries.

[b] Routine for certain age groups and risk factors, selective for general travellers.

[c] No longer routine in most industrialized countries.

[d] These vaccines are also included in the routine immunization programme in several countries.

Some polio-free countries may also require travellers from polio-endemic countries to be immunized against polio in order to obtain an entry visa, e.g. Saudi Arabia. Updates are available on http://www.who.int/wer

Travellers should be provided with a written record of all vaccines administered (patient-retained record), preferably using the international vaccination certificate (which is required in the case of yellow fever vaccination).

Vaccines for routine use

Recommendations on vaccines for routine use are provided by WHO in regularly updated vaccine position papers: http://www.who.int/immunization/documents/positionpapers_intro/en/index.html

Since the information provided in this chapter is limited, readers are encouraged to refer to the WHO vaccine position papers as well as to national guidelines on routine vaccinations. It is recommended that travellers ensure that all routine vaccinations are up to date. Information on safety of routine vaccines can be found at: http://www.who.int/vaccine_safety/en/

DIPHTHERIA/TETANUS/PERTUSSIS

DIPHTHERIA

Disease

Diphtheria is a bacterial disease caused by *Corynebacterium diphtheriae*. The infection commonly affects the throat and may lead to obstruction of the airways and death. Exotoxin-induced damage occurs to organs such as the heart. Nasal diphtheria may be mild, and chronic carriage of the organism frequently occurs; asymptomatic infections are common. Transmission is from person to person, through droplets and close physical contact, and is increased in overcrowded and poor socioeconomic conditions. A cutaneous form of diphtheria is common in tropical countries and may be important in transmission of the infection.

Occurrence

Diphtheria is found worldwide, although it is not common in industrialized countries because of long-standing routine use of DTP vaccine. Large epidemics occurred in several east European countries in the 1990s.

Risk for travellers

Potentially life-threatening illness and severe, lifelong complications are possible in incompletely immunized individuals. Diphtheria is more frequent in parts of the world where vaccination levels are low.

Vaccine

All travellers should be up to date with the vaccine, which is usually given as "triple vaccine" – DTP (diphtheria/tetanus/pertussis). After the initial course of three doses, additional doses may be given as DT until 7 years of age, after which a vaccine with reduced diphtheria content (Td) is given. Since both tetanus tox-oid (see below) and diphtheria toxoid can reasonably be given on a booster basis about every 10 years, there is no reason to use monovalent diphtheria vaccine. In some countries, adult boosters that contain acellular pertussis (dTaP) are being introduced.

TETANUS

Disease

Tetanus is acquired through environmental exposure to the spores of *Clostridium tetani*, which are present in soil worldwide. The disease is caused by the action of a potent neurotoxin produced by the bacterium in dead tissue (e.g. dirty wounds). Clinical symptoms of tetanus are muscle spasms, initially of the muscles of mastication causing trismus or "lockjaw", which results in a characteristic facial expression – risus sardonicus. Trismus can be followed by sustained spasm of the back muscles (opisthotonus) and by spasms of other muscles. Finally, mild external stimuli may trigger generalized, tetanic seizures, which contribute to the serious complications of tetanus (dysphagia, aspiration pneumonia) and lead to death unless intense supportive treatment is rapidly initiated.

Occurrence

Dirty wounds can become infected with the spores of *Clostridium tetani* anywhere in the world.

Risk for travellers

Every traveller should be fully protected against tetanus. Almost any form of injury, from a simple laceration to a motor-vehicle accident, can expose the individual to the spores.

Vaccine

Tetanus toxoid vaccine is available as single toxoid (TT), combined with diphtheria toxoid (DT) or low-dose diphtheria toxoid (Td), and combined with diphtheria and pertussis vaccines (whole pertussis wP or acellular pertussis aP) (DTwP, DTaP, or dTaP). Vaccines containing DT are used for children under 7 years of age and dT-containing vaccines for those aged 7 years and over. Vaccine combinations containing diphtheria toxoid (D or d) and tetanus toxoid, rather than tetanus toxoid alone, should be used when immunization against tetanus is indicated.

A childhood immunization schedule of 5 doses is recommended. The primary series of 3 doses of DTP (DTwP or DTaP) should be given in infancy, with a booster dose of a tetanus toxoid-containing vaccine ideally at age 4–7 years and another booster in adolescence, e.g. at age 12–15 years. For adult travellers, an extra tetanus toxoid-containing dose will provide additional assurance of long-lasting, possibly lifelong, protection.

All travellers should be up to date with the vaccine before departure. The type of tetanus prophylaxis that is required following injury depends on the nature of the lesion and the history of previous immunizations. However, no booster is needed if the last dose of tetanus vaccine was given less than 5 (for dirty wounds) to 10 years (for clean wounds) previously.

PERTUSSIS

Disease

Pertussis (whooping cough) is a highly contagious acute bacterial disease involving the respiratory tract and caused by *Bordetella pertussis*. It is transmitted by direct contact with airborne discharges from the respiratory mucous membranes of infected persons. It causes a severe cough of several weeks' duration with a characteristic whoop, often with cyanosis and vomiting. In young infants, the cough may be absent and disease may manifest with spells of apnoea. Although pertussis can occur at any age, most serious cases and fatalities are observed in early infancy and mainly in developing countries. Major complications include pneumonia, encephalitis and malnutrition (due to repeated vomiting). Vaccination is the most rational approach to pertussis control.

Occurrence

Recent estimates from WHO suggest that about 17.6 million cases of pertussis occurred worldwide in 2003, 90% of which were in developing countries, and that some 279 000 patients died from this disease.

Risk for travellers

Unprotected infants are at high risk, but all children and young adults are at risk if they are not fully immunized. Exposure to pertussis is greater in developing countries.

Vaccine

All travellers should be up to date with the vaccine. Both whole-cell (wP) and acellular (aP) pertussis vaccines provide excellent protection. For several decades, wP vaccines have been widely used in national childhood vaccination programmes; aP vaccines, which cause fewer adverse effects, have been developed and are now being licensed in several countries. Both wP and aP are usually administered in combination with diphtheria and tetanus toxoids (DTwP or DTaP). Three doses are required for initial protection. Protection declines with time and probably lasts only a few years. A booster dose administered 1–6 years after the primary series is warranted. Some countries now offer an adult/adolescent booster, in particular to health care workers and young parents. Only aP or dTaP vaccines are used for vaccination of older children and adults.

HAEMOPHILUS INFLUENZAE TYPE B

Disease

Haemophilus influenzae type b (Hib) is a common cause of bacterial pneumonia and meningitis and of a number of other serious and potentially life-threatening conditions, including epiglottitis, osteomyelitis, septic arthritis and sepsis in infants and older children.

Occurrence

Hib is estimated to cause at least 3 million cases of serious disease and hundreds of thousands of deaths annually, worldwide. Rarely occurring in infants under 3 months or after the age of 6 years, the disease burden is highest between 4 and 18 months of age. Hib is the dominant cause of sporadic (non-epidemic) bacterial meningitis in this age group, and is frequently associated with severe neurological sequelae despite prompt and adequate antibiotic treatment. In developing countries, it is estimated that 2–3 million cases of Hib pneumonia occur each year. The disease has practically disappeared in countries where routine vaccination of children is carried out.

Risk for travellers

All unprotected children are at risk at least up to the age of 5 years.

Vaccine

All children who are not up to date with this vaccine should be offered it. Conjugate Hib vaccines have dramatically reduced the incidence of Hib meningitis in infants and of nasopharyngeal colonization by Hib. The vaccine is often given as a combined preparation with DTP or poliomyelitis vaccine in routine immunization programmes, but is available as a single antigen preparation for use in children who did not receive the vaccine as part of routine immunization. Hib vaccine is not yet used routinely in many developing countries where there is continuing high prevalence of the disease.

HEPATITIS B

Disease and occurrence

See Chapter 5.

Risk for travellers

The risk depends on (1) the prevalence of HBV infection in the country of destination, (2) the extent of direct contact with blood or body fluids or of sexual contact with potentially infected persons, and (3) the duration and type of travel. Principal risky activities include health care (medical, dental, laboratory or other) that entails direct exposure to human blood or body fluids; receipt of a transfusion of blood that has not been tested for HBV; and dental, medical or other exposure to needles (e.g. acupuncture, piercing, tattooing or injecting drug use) that have not been appropriately sterilized. In addition, in less developed countries, transmission from HBV-positive to HBV-susceptible individuals may occur through direct contact between open skin lesions following a penetrating bite or scratch.

The vaccine should be considered for virtually all non-immune individuals travelling to areas with moderate to high risk of infection. It can be administered to infants from birth.

Vaccine

Hepatitis B vaccine produced both from plasma and by recombinant DNA technology (usually in yeast) is available; the two types are equally safe and effective. Three doses of vaccine constitute the complete series; the first two doses are usually given 1 month apart, with the third dose 1–12 months later.

Immunization provides protection for at least 15 years and, according to current scientific evidence, probably for life. Because of the prolonged incubation period of hepatitis B, some protection will be afforded to most travellers following the second dose given before travel, provided that the final dose is given upon return. The standard schedule of administration is three doses, given as follows: day 0; 1 month; 6–12 months.

A rapid schedule of administration of monovalent hepatitis B vaccine has been proposed by the manufacturer as follows: day 0; 1 month; 2 months. An additional dose is given 6-12 months after the first dose.

A very rapid schedule of administration of monovalent hepatitis B vaccine has been proposed as follows: day 0; 7 days; 21 days. An additional dose is given at 12 months.

A combination vaccine that provides protection against both hepatitis A and hepatitis B may be considered for travellers potentially exposed to both organisms. This inactivated vaccine is administered as follows: day 0; 1 month; 6 months. A rapid schedule at day 0, 1 month and 2 months, with an additional dose at 12 months, has been proposed by the vaccine manufacturer, as well as a very rapid schedule with administration at day 0, day 7 and day 21 with a booster dose at 12 months.

HUMAN PAPILLOMAVIRUS

Disease

Human papillomavirus (HPV) is a family of viruses that are very common all over the world. Although most HPV infections cause no symptoms and are self-limited, persistent genital HPV infection can cause cervical cancer in women (as well as other types of anogenital cancers, head and neck cancers, and genital warts in both men and women).

Occurrence

HPV is common worldwide and estimated to cause more than half a million new cancers every year and 274 000 deaths (2002 estimate), most of which affect women in developing countries.

Risk for travellers

Travel itself does not increase the risk of exposure. Transmission of HPV is most commonly through sexual activity: condoms may not offer complete protection. In 2006, a vaccine targeting four HPV genotypes (including those that are responsible for 70% of cervical cancer cases worldwide) was licensed in the USA and in several other countries, and another vaccine is expected to be licensed soon. The vaccine is intended for use primarily in girls and young women for the prevention of diseases caused by the HPV genotypes included in the vaccine. Over the next few years, HPV vaccination will be introduced into the immunization schedules of several countries. Travellers are advised to check with the relevant health authorities regarding national recommendations and the availability of HPV vaccination in their country.

INFLUENZA

Disease and occurrence

See Chapter 5.

Risk for travellers

In the tropics, influenza can occur throughout the year. In the southern hemisphere, peak activity occurs between April and September and in the northern hemisphere between November and March. Influenza transmission may be enhanced in crowded conditions associated with air travel, cruise ships and tour groups. Elderly people and individuals with respiratory and cardiac disease, diabetes mellitus or any immunosuppressive condition are particularly at risk of more severe disease. The impact of an attack of influenza during travel can range from highly inconvenient to life-threatening.

Vaccine

Influenza viruses constantly evolve, with rapid changes in their antigenic characteristics. To be effective, influenza vaccines need to stimulate immunity to the principal strains of virus circulating at the time. In a very limited number of countries, a live vaccine is being used. The internationally available vaccines contain three inactivated viral strains, with the composition being modified every 6 months to ensure protection against the strains prevailing in each influenza season. Since the antigenic changes in circulating influenza viruses occur very rapidly, there may be significant differences between prevailing strains during the influenza seasons of the northern and southern hemispheres, which occur at different times of the year. Vaccine composition is therefore adjusted for the hemisphere in which the vaccine will be used. Thus, a vaccine obtainable in one hemisphere may offer only partial protection against influenza infection in the other.

Travellers belonging to the high-risk groups for influenza should be regularly vaccinated each year. Those travelling from one hemisphere to the other shortly before, or early during, the influenza season should obtain vaccination for the opposite hemisphere in a travel clinic or – if not available – arrange vaccination as soon as possible after arriving at the travel destination.

One dose is given i.m. for individuals over 9 years of age. Two doses at least 4 weeks apart for immunocompromised people and for children aged 6 months – 9 years; those aged 3–36 months should receive half the adult vaccines injections. Mild local and/or systemic reactions are common. Vaccination is contraindicated in case of egg allergy.

MEASLES

Disease

Measles is a highly contagious infection; before vaccines became available this disease had affected most people by the time of adolescence. In 2002, measles still affected about 30 million persons, and the number of global measles deaths was estimated to be 610 000. Common complications include middle-ear infection and pneumonia. Transmission, which is primarily by large respiratory droplets, increases during the late winter and early spring in temperate climates, and after the rainy season in tropical climates.

Occurrence

Measles occurs worldwide in a seasonal pattern. However, following the introduction of large-scale measles immunization, far fewer cases now occur in industrialized countries and indigenous transmission has virtually stopped in the Americas. Epidemics may still occur every 2 or 3 years in areas where there is low vaccine coverage. In countries where measles has been largely eliminated, cases imported from other countries remain an important continuing source of infection.

Risk for travellers

Travellers who are not fully immunized against measles are at risk when visiting countries or areas where vaccine coverage is incomplete.

Vaccine

The measles/mumps/rubella triple (MMR) or measles/rubella (MR) vaccine is given in many countries instead of monovalent measles vaccine. In industrialized countries, measles vaccination is usually given at the age of 12–15 months, when seroconversion rates in excess of 90% are expected. In most developing countries, high attack rates and serious disease among infants necessitate early vaccination, usually at 9 months of age, despite the relatively low (80–85%) seroconversion rates following vaccination in this age group. To ensure optimum population immunity, all children should be given a second opportunity for measles immunization. Although generally administered at school entry (age 4–6 years), the second dose may be given as early as one month following the first dose, depending on the local programmatic and epidemiological situation.

Special attention must be paid to all children and adolescent/young adult travellers who have not been vaccinated against measles at the appropriate time. Measles is still common in many countries and travel in densely populated areas may favour transmission. For infants travelling to countries where measles is endemic, a dose of vaccine may be given as early as 6 months of age. However, children who receive the first dose between 6 and 8 months should subsequently receive the two doses according to the national schedule. Older children or adults who did not receive the two lifetime doses should consider this before travel.

It is generally recommended that individuals with a moderate degree of immune deficiency receive the vaccine if there is even a low risk of contracting measles infection from the community. There is a low level of risk in using measles vaccine in immunocompromised HIV-infected individuals. Where the risk of contracting measles infection is negligible, physicians who are able to monitor immune status, for instance CD4 counts, may prefer to avoid the use of measles vaccine.

MUMPS

Disease

Mumps, or parotitis epidemica, is a viral infection that primarily affects the salivary glands. Although mumps is mostly a mild childhood disease, the virus may also affect adults, in whom complications such as meningitis and orchitis are relatively common. Encephalitis and permanent neurological sequelae are rare complications of mumps.

Occurrence

In most parts of the world, annual mumps incidence is in the range of 100–1000 per 100 000 population, with epidemic peaks every 2–5 years. Peak incidence is found among children aged 5–9 years. Natural infection with mumps virus is thought to confer lifelong protection.

Risk for travellers

Travellers who are not fully immunized against mumps are at risk when visiting endemic countries.

Vaccine

The mumps vaccine is usually given in combination with measles and rubella vaccine (MMR). Different attenuated strains of the mumps virus are used for the production of live mumps vaccines, all of which are considered safe and efficacious, except for the Rubini strain. In order to avoid possible interference with persistent maternal antibodies, the recommended one dose of the vaccine is usually given at 12–18 months of age. A single dose of mumps vaccine, either as single antigen or in combination, has a protective efficacy of 90–96%, and the second dose given in some countries at age 4–6 years provides protection to most individuals who do not respond to the first.

RUBELLA

Disease

Rubella occurs worldwide and is normally a mild childhood disease. However, infection during early pregnancy may cause fetal death or congenital rubella syndrome (CRS) which is characterized by multiple defects, particularly of the brain, heart, eyes and ears. CRS is an important cause of hearing and visual impairment and mental retardation in countries where acquired rubella infection has not been controlled or eliminated.

Occurrence

Although the worldwide burden of CRS is not well characterized, it is estimated that more than 100 000 cases occur each year in developing countries alone.

Risk for travellers

Travellers who are not immunized against rubella may be at risk when visiting countries where the vaccine coverage is suboptimal. Particular attention should be paid to ensuring protection of women who may become pregnant during the period of travel.

Vaccine

The internationally licensed rubella vaccines, based on live attenuated RA 27/3 strain of the rubella virus and propagated in human diploid cells, have proved to be safe and efficacious. Following well designed and implemented programmes using such vaccines, rubella and CRS have almost disappeared from many countries. Other attenuated vaccine strains are available in Japan and China.

Rubella vaccine is commercially available in a monovalent form, in a bivalent combination with either measles or mumps vaccine, and in the trivalent measles/mumps/rubella (MMR) vaccine. Rubella vaccination of pregnant women should be avoided, and pregnancy should be avoided within one month of receiving the vaccine.

PNEUMOCOCCAL DISEASE

Disease

The term "pneumococcal disease" refers to a group of clinical conditions caused by the bacterium *Streptococcus pneumoniae*. Invasive pneumococcal infections include pneumonia, meningitis and febrile bacteraemia; the common non-invasive conditions include otitis media, sinusitis and bronchitis. Infection is acquired by direct person-to-person contact via respiratory droplets or oral contact. There are many healthy, asymptomatic carriers of the bacteria, but there is no animal reservoir or insect vector.

Several chronic conditions predispose to serious pneumococcal disease (see below). Increasing pneumococcal resistance to antibiotics underlines the importance of vaccination.

Occurrence

Pneumococcal diseases are a worldwide public health problem. *S. pneumoniae* is the leading cause of severe pneumonia in children under 5 years of age, causing more than 700 000 deaths each year, mainly in developing countries. In industrialized countries, most pneumococcal disease occurs in the elderly.

Risk for travellers

While travel itself does not increase the risk of acquiring pneumococcal infection, access to optimal health care may be limited during travel, increasing the risk of poor outcomes should disease occur. Certain conditions predispose to complications of pneumococcal infections, including sickle-cell disease, other haemoglobinopathies, chronic renal failure, chronic liver disease, immunosuppression after organ transplantation and other etiological factors, asplenia and dysfunctional spleen, leaks of cerebrospinal fluid, diabetes mellitus and HIV infection. Elderly individuals, especially those over the age of 65 years, are also at increased risk for pneumococcal disease. Pneumococcal vaccine is recommended for travellers who belong to these high-risk groups.

Vaccine

The current 23-valent polysaccharide vaccine represents pneumococcal serotypes that are responsible for 90% of pneumococcal infections and is immunogenic in those over 2 years of age. Children under 2 years of age and immunocompromised individuals do not respond well to the vaccine. Vaccination provides a relative protection against invasive pneumococcal disease in healthy elderly individuals. Pneumococcal polysaccharide vaccine is recommended for selected groups, over the age of 2 years, at increased risk of pneumococcal disease. In some countries, such as the USA, routine vaccination is recommended for everyone aged over 65 years.

A conjugate vaccine containing seven serotypes of the pneumococcus is now available and is safe and immunogenic also in infants and children under 2 years. This vaccine is recommended as part of routine immunization in infants in some countries and in children at risk in others. It is advisable that children be up to date with immunization, as per the national recommendations, before undertaking travel.

POLIOMYELITIS

Disease

Poliomyelitis is a disease of the central nervous system caused by three closely related enteroviruses, poliovirus types 1, 2 and 3. The virus is spread predominantly by the faecal–oral route, although rare outbreaks caused by contaminated food or water have occurred. After the virus enters the mouth, the primary site of infection is the intestine, although the virus can also be found in the pharynx. Poliomyelitis is also known as "infantile paralysis" because it most frequently caused paralysis in infants and young children in the pre-vaccine era in industrialized countries. In developing countries, 60–70% of cases currently occur in children under 3 years of age and 90% in children under 5 years of age. The resulting paralysis is permanent, although some recovery of function is possible. There is no cure.

Occurrence

Significant progress has been made towards global eradication of poliomyelitis. More than 125 countries were endemic for polio in 1988; by 2006, only 4 countries – Afghanistan, India, Nigeria and Pakistan (see map), where wild poliovirus transmission has never been interrupted – remained endemic. A number of previously polio-free countries have been affected by wild-virus importation that has resulted in subsequent outbreaks, e.g. Namibia – a popular country for tourists – in the summer of 2006. Until all countries have stopped wild poliovirus transmission, all areas remain at high risk of importations and even of the re-establishment of endemic transmission.

Risks associated with international travel

The consequences of polio infection are life-threatening or crippling. Infection and paralysis may occur in non-immune individuals and are by no means confined to infants. Infected travellers are potent vectors for transmission and possible reintroduction of the virus into polio-free zones, now that worldwide eradication is near. Until the disease has been certified as eradicated globally, the risks of acquiring polio (for travellers to infected areas), and of re-infection of polio-free areas (by travellers from infected areas), remain. Travellers to and from endemic countries should be fully protected by vaccination.

Vaccine

All travellers to and from polio-infected areas should be up to date with vaccination against poliomyelitis according to national immunization policy. There are two types of vaccine: inactivated (IPV), which is given by injection, and oral (OPV). OPV is composed of the three types of live attenuated polioviruses. Because of the low cost and ease of administration of the vaccine and its superiority in conferring intestinal immunity, OPV has been the vaccine of choice for controlling epidemic poliomyelitis in many countries. On very rare occasions (2–4 cases per million births per year) OPV causes vaccine-associated paralytic poliomyelitis (VAPP). The risk of VAPP is higher with the first dose of OPV than with subsequent doses. VAPP is more common in individuals who are immunocompromised, for whom IPV is the vaccine of choice.

Most industrialized countries use IPV, either as the sole vaccine against poliomyelitis or in schedules combined with OPV. Although IPV suppresses pharyngeal excretion of wild poliovirus, this vaccine has only limited effects in reducing intestinal excretion of poliovirus. For unvaccinated older children and adults, the second dose is given 1–2 months, and the third 6–12 months, after the first dose. A booster dose is recommended after 4–6 years. IPV is also the vaccine of choice for travellers with no history of OPV use, as well as for immunocompromised individuals and their contacts and family members.

For those who have received three or more doses of OPV in the past, it is advisable to offer another dose of polio vaccine as a once-only dose to those travelling to endemic areas of the world. Any unimmunized individuals intending to travel to such areas require a complete course of vaccine. Countries differ in recommending IPV or OPV in these circumstances: the advantage of IPV is that any risk of VAPP is avoided, but this vaccine is more expensive and may not prevent faecal excretion of the virus.

In order to limit further international spread of wild poliovirus to polio-free areas, travellers from an infected country or area should have a full course of vaccination against polio before leaving their country of residence, with a minimum one dose of OPV before departure. Some polio-free countries may also require travellers from endemic countries to be immunized against polio in order to obtain an entry visa.

ROTAVIRUS

Disease

Rotavirus causes an acute gastroenteritis in infants and young children and is associated with profuse watery diarrhoea, projectile vomiting and fever. Rapid dehydration can occur, especially in very young infants, requiring rehydration therapy. The virus is transmitted via the faecal–oral route and by direct person-to-person spread, although a respiratory mode of transmission has been proposed also. It replicates in the enterocytes of the small intestine, causing extensive damage to the microvilli that results in malabsorption and loss of fluids and electrolytes.

Occurrence

Rotavirus is found worldwide. The virus is ubiquitous, infecting a large proportion of young children by their second or third birthday. Re-infection of older children and adults is common, although the infection is usually sub-clinical.

Risk for travellers

The potential risk for travellers is extremely limited since most individuals will have good immunity through repeated exposures early in life.

Vaccine

Two live, attenuated, oral rotavirus vaccines are internationally licensed and routine childhood vaccination has been initiated in a number of countries. However, vaccination is not currently recommended for travellers or older children outside the routine childhood immunization schedule.

TUBERCULOSIS

Disease and occurrence

See Chapter 5.

Risk for travellers

Most travellers are at low risk for tuberculosis (TB). The risk for long-term travellers (>3 months) in a country with a higher incidence of TB than their own may be comparable to the risk for local residents. Living conditions, as well as duration of travel and purpose of travel, e.g. emergency relief, are important in determining the risk of infection: high-risk settings include impoverished communities, areas experiencing civil unrest or war, refugee areas, health facilities, prisons and shelters for the homeless. Persons with HIV infection are at higher risk of TB.

Vaccine

All versions of the BCG vaccine are based on live, attenuated mycobacterial strains descended from the original, attenuated bacillus Calmette-Guérin. The vaccine is administered intradermally and can be given simultaneously with other childhood vaccines. BCG vaccine is contraindicated for persons with severely impaired immunity, including individuals with HIV infection.

BCG vaccine is of very limited use for travellers. In the first year of life it provides good protection against forms of TB associated with haematogenous spread (miliary TB and meningitis). In countries with high TB prevalence, infants are generally immunized with a single dose of BCG as soon after birth as possible. Other protective benefits of the vaccine are uncertain. BCG should be considered for infants travelling from an area of low incidence to one of high incidence.

Many industrialized countries with a low incidence of TB have ceased giving BCG routinely to neonates.

Booster doses of BCG are not recommended by WHO.

VARICELLA

Disease and occurence

The causative pathogen is the varicella zoster virus (VZV). Varicella (chickenpox) is an acute, highly contagious disease with worldwide distribution. In temperate climates most cases occur before the age of 10 years. The epidemiology is less well understood in tropical areas, where a relatively large proportion of adults in some countries are seronegative.

Transmission is via droplets, aerosol or direct contact, and patients are usually contagious from a few days before rash onset until the rash has crusted over. While mostly a mild disorder in childhood, varicella tends to be more severe in adults. It is characterized by an itchy, vesicular rash, usually starting on the scalp and face, and initially accompanied by fever and malaise. As the rash gradually spreads to the trunk and extremities, the first vesicles dry out. It normally takes about 7–10 days for all crusts to disappear. The disease may be fatal, especially in neonates and immunocompromised persons. Complications include VZV-induced pneumonitis or encephalitis and invasive group A streptococcal infections. Following infection, the virus remains latent in neural ganglia; upon subsequent reactivation, VZV may cause zoster (shingles), a disease affecting mainly immunocompromised persons and the elderly.

Risk for travellers

In several industrialized countries, varicella vaccines have been introduced into the childhood immunization programmes. Most adult travellers from temperate climates are immune (as a result of either natural disease or immunization). Adult travellers without a history of varicella who travel from tropical countries to temperate climates may be at increased risk.

Vaccine

Various formulations of the live attenuated vaccine, based on the so-called Oka strain of VZV, are in use. Some formulations are approved for use at 9 months of age and older. Following a single dose, seroconversion occurs in about 95% of healthy children. From a logistic as well as an epidemiological point of view, the optimal age for varicella vaccination is 12–24 months. In Japan and several other countries, 1 dose of the vaccine is considered sufficient, regardless of age. In the United States, 2 doses, 4–8 weeks apart, are recommended for adolescents and adults. In a few cases (less than 5%) vaccinees experience a mild varicella-like disease with rash within 4 weeks. Contraindications to varicella vaccine are pregnancy (because of a theoretical risk to the fetus; pregnancy should be avoided for 4 weeks following vaccination), ongoing severe illness, a history of anaphylactic reactions to any component of the vaccine, and immunosuppression.

Vaccines for selective use

Vaccines in this section need be offered only to travellers who are going to certain specific destinations. The decision to recommend a vaccine will depend on a travel risk assessment for the individual.

CHOLERA

Disease and occurrence

See Chapter 5.

Risk for travellers

Travellers are not at significant risk from cholera provided that simple precautions are taken to avoid potentially contaminated food and water. Vaccination is of questionable benefit to general tourist travellers, for whom the risk is very low, and is therefore recommended only for individuals at increased risk of exposure, particularly emergency relief and health workers in refugee situations.

Cholera vaccination is not required as a condition of entry to any country.

Vaccine

Although two new cholera vaccines (live and killed), given orally, are safe and effective and have been licensed in a limited number of countries, the live vaccine is currently no longer available commercially. The inactivated or killed vaccine confers high-grade (85–90%) protection for 6 months after the second dose, to be given at least one week after the first. After 3 years, protection remains as high as 62% in vaccine recipients over 5 years of age.

Precautions and contraindications

None.

Type of vaccine:	Killed oral
Number of doses:	Two, at least 1 week apart (killed vaccine)
Contraindications:	Hypersensitivity to previous dose
Adverse reactions:	Mild gastrointestinal disturbances reported
Before departure:	3 weeks (killed vaccine)
Consider for:	Travellers at high risk (e.g. emergency or relief workers)
Special precautions:	None

HEPATITIS A

Disease and occurrence

Although hepatitis A is rarely fatal in children and young adults, most infected adults and some older children become ill and are unable to work for several weeks or months. The case-fatality rate exceeds 2% among those over 40 years of age and may be 4% for those aged 60 years or more. (See also Chapter 5.)

Risk for travellers

The vaccine should be considered for all travellers to areas with moderate to high risk of infection, and those at high risk of acquiring the disease should be strongly encouraged to be vaccinated regardless of where they travel.

People born and raised in developing countries, and those born before 1945 in industrialized countries, have often been infected in childhood and are likely to be immune. For such individuals, it may be cost-effective to test for antibodies to hepatitis A virus (anti-HAV) so that unnecessary vaccination can be avoided.

Vaccine

Current hepatitis A vaccines, all of which based on inactivated (killed) virus, are safe and highly effective. Anti-HAV antibodies are detectable by 2 weeks after administration of the first dose of vaccine. The second dose – given at least 6 months, and usually 6–24 months, after the first dose – is necessary to promote long-term protection. Results from mathematical models indicate that, after completion of the primary series, anti-HAV antibodies probably persist for 25 years or more. Booster doses are not recommended. Serological testing to assess antibody levels after vaccination is not indicated. Given the long incubation period of hepatitis A (average 2–4 weeks), the vaccine can be administered up to the day of departure and still protect travellers. The use of immune globulin is now virtually obsolete for the purposes of travel prophylaxis.

A combination hepatitis A/typhoid vaccine is available for those exposed to waterborne diseases. The vaccine is administered as a single dose and confers high levels of protection against both diseases. A second dose of hepatitis A vaccine is needed 6–24 months later and boosters of typhoid vaccine should be given at 3-yearly intervals.

A combination vaccine that provides protection against both hepatitis A and hepatitis B may be considered for travellers who may be exposed to both organisms. Primary immunization with the combined hepatitis A and B vaccine consist of three doses, given on a schedule of 0, 1 and 6 months. According to the manufacturer's instructions, this combination vaccine may also be administered on days 0, 7 and 21, with a booster dose at 12 months.

Precautions and contraindications

Minor local and systemic reactions are fairly common. Minimum age is 1 year.

Type of vaccine:	Inactivated, given i.m.
Number of doses:	Two
Schedule:	Second dose 6–24 months after the first
Booster:	May not be necessary
Contraindications:	Hypersensitivity to previous dose
Adverse reactions:	Mild local reaction of short duration, mild systemic reaction
Before departure:	Protection 2–4 weeks after first dose
Recommended for:	All non-immune travellers to endemic areas
Special precautions:	None

JAPANESE ENCEPHALITIS

Disease and occurrence

See Chapter 5.

Risk for travellers

Japanese encephalitis (JE) is the leading cause of viral encephalitis in Asia and occurs in almost all Asian countries (see map). Its incidence has been declining in Japan and the Korean peninsula and in some regions of China, but is increasing in Bangladesh, India, Nepal, Pakistan, northern Thailand and Viet Nam. Transmission occurs principally in rural agricultural locations where flooding irrigation is practised – some of which may be near or within urban centres. Transmission is seasonal and mainly related to the rainy season in south-east Asia. In the temperate regions of China, Japan, the Korean peninsula and eastern parts of the Russian Federation, transmission occurs mainly during the summer and autumn. Vaccination is not recommended for all travellers to Asia because of the low incidence of the disease in travellers and potential (although rare) adverse events: it should be based on individual risk assessment, taking into account the season, the type of accommodation and the duration of exposure, as well as the travel itinerary. The risk to short-term travellers and those who travel mainly to urban areas is very low. Vaccination is recommended for travellers with extensive outdoor exposure (camping, hiking, bicycle tours, outdoor occupational activities, in particular in areas where flooding irrigation is practised) in rural areas of an endemic region during the transmission season. It is also recommended for expatriates living in endemic areas through a transmission season or longer.

Vaccine

Three types of JE vaccine are currently in large-scale production and use: inactivated mouse-brain-derived vaccine (IMB), cell-culture-derived inactivated vaccine and cell-culture-derived live attenuated SA 14-14-2 vaccine. At present, the IMB vaccine is the most widely available commercially, but its production may cease in the future.

Precautions and contraindications

A hypersensitivity reaction to a previous dose is a contraindication. The live attenuated vaccine should be avoided in pregnancy unless the likely risk favours its administration. Rare, but serious, neurological side-effects attributed to IMB vaccine have been reported from endemic as well as non-endemic regions. Allergic reactions to components of the vaccine occur occasionally. As such reactions may occur within 2 weeks of administration, it is advisable to ensure that the complete course of vaccine is administered well in advance of departure.

Type of vaccine:	Inactivated mouse-brain-derived or live attenuated
Schedule:	For the inactivated vaccine: 3 doses at days 0, 7 and 28; or 2 doses given preferably 4 weeks apart (0.5 or 1.0 ml for adults, 0.25 or 0.5 ml for children depending on the vaccines)
	For the live attenuated SA14-14-2 vaccine equally good protection is achieved with a single dose followed, as required, with a single booster dose given at an interval of about 1 year
Booster:	After 1 year and then 3-yearly (for IMB only) when continued protection is requireda
Contraindications:	Hypersensitivity to a previous dose of vaccine, pregnancy and immunosuppression (live vaccine)
Adverse reactions:	Occasional mild local or systemic reaction; occasional severe reaction with generalized urticaria, hypotension and collapse
Before departure:	Inactivated vaccine, at least two doses before departure. Live attenuated vaccine, one dose is enough

[a] The duration of immunity after serial booster doses in adult travellers has not been well established for the mouse-brain-derived vaccine. For children aged 1–3 years, the mouse-brain-derived vaccine provides adequate protection throughout childhood following two primary doses 4 weeks apart and boosters after 1 year and subsequently at 3-yearly intervals until the age of 10–15 years.

MENINGOCOCCAL DISEASE

Disease and occurrence

See Chapter 5.

Risk for travellers

Vaccination should be considered for travellers to countries where outbreaks of meningococcal disease are known to occur.

- Travellers to industrialized countries are exposed to the possibility of sporadic cases. Outbreaks of meningococcal C disease occur in schools, colleges, military barracks and other places where large numbers of adolescents and young adults congregate.

- Travellers to the sub-Saharan meningitis belt may be exposed to outbreaks of serogroup A disease with comparatively very high incidence rates during the dry season (December–June). Long-term travellers living in close contact with the indigenous population may be at greater risk of infection.

- Pilgrims to Mecca are at risk. The tetravalent vaccine, (A, C, Y, W-135) is currently required by Saudi Arabia for pilgrims visiting Mecca for the Hajj (annual pilgrimage) or for the Umrah. Outbreaks of meningococcal disease have affected these pilgrims in the past, involving serogroup A in 1987 and both serogroups A and W135 more recently.

Vaccine

Polysaccharide vacnes

Internationally marketed meningococcal polysaccharide vaccines are either bivalent (A and C) or tetravalent (A, C, Y and W-135).The vaccines are purified, heat-stable, lyophilized capsular polysaccharides from meningococci of the respective serogroups.

Both group A and group C vaccines have documented short-term efficacy levels of 85–100% in older children and adults. However, group C vaccines do not prevent disease in children under 2 years of age, and the efficacy of group A vaccine in children under 1 year of age is unclear. Group Y and W-135 polysaccharides have been shown to be immunogenic only in children over 2 years of age.

A protective antibody response occurs within 10 days of vaccination. In school-children and adults, the bivalent and tetravalent polysaccharide vaccines appear to provide protection for at least 3 years, but in children under 4 years the levels of specific antibodies decline rapidly after 2–3 years.

The currently available bivalent and tetravalent meningococcal vaccines are recommended for immunization of specific risk groups as well as for large-scale immunization, as appropriate, for the control of meningococcal outbreaks caused by vaccine-preventable serogroups (A and C, or A, C, Y, W-135 respectively). Travellers who have access to the tetravalent polysaccharide vaccine (A, C, Y, W-135) should opt for this rather than the bivalent vaccine because of the additional protection against groups Y and W-135.

These vaccines do not provide any protection against group B meningococci, which are the leading cause of endemic meningococcal disease in some countries.

Conjugate vaccines

A T-cell-dependent immune response is achieved through conjugation of the polysaccharide to a protein carrier. Conjugate vaccines are therefore associated with an increased immunogenicity among infants and prolonged duration of protection.

Monovalent serogroup C conjugate vaccines were first licensed for use in 1999 and are now incorporated in national vaccination programmes in an increasing number of countries. In contrast to group C polysaccharide vaccines, the group C conjugate vaccine elicits adequate antibody responses and immunological memory even in infants who are vaccinated at 2, 3 and 4 months of age.

More recently, a tetravalent conjugate vaccine (A, C, Y, W-135) has been licensed in a limited number of countries.

Precautions and contraindications

The internationally available polysaccharide vaccines are safe, and significant systemic reactions have been extremely rare. The most common adverse reactions are erythema and slight pain at the site of injection for 1–2 days. Fever exceeding 38.5 °C occurs in up to 2% of vaccinees. No significant change in safety or reactogenicity has been observed when the different group-specific polysaccharides are combined into bivalent or tetravalent meningococcal vaccines. Cross-protection does not occur and travellers already immunized with conjugate vaccine against serogroup C are not protected against other serogroups.

Type of vaccine:	Purified bacterial capsular polysaccharide meningococcal vaccine (bivalent or tetravalent)
Number of doses:	One
Duration of protection:	3–5 years
Contraindications:	Serious adverse reaction to previous dose
Adverse reactions:	Occasional mild local reactions, rarely, fever
Before departure:	2 weeks
Consider for:	All travellers to countries in the sub-Saharan meningitis belt and to areas with current epidemics; college students at risk from endemic disease; Hajj and Umrah pilgrims (mandatory)
Special precautions:	Children under 2 years of age are not protected by the vaccine

RABIES

Disease and occurrence

See Chapter 5

Risk for travellers

The risk to travellers in rabies-endemic areas (see map, or www.who.int/rabnet) is proportional to their contact with potentially rabid animals. For instance, it is estimated that 13% of visitors to one country in South-East Asia come into contact with local animals. Dogs, both owned and ownerless, are very common, with an estimated 1:10 ratio of dogs to humans in most developing countries. An average of 100 suspected rabid dog bites per 100 000 inhabitants are reported in endemic countries with dog rabies. According to a recent survey conducted in India, 1.6% of the total population received a dog bite during a 12-month period. Veterinarians and people working with dogs are at the greatest risk. Most travellers in tourist resorts are at very low risk. There is a greater risk for children, however, who may have more contact with animals and may not report suspect incidents. It is prudent to avoid walking in areas where dogs roam. Following suspect contact, especially bites or scratches, medical advice should be sought at once at a competent medical centre, ideally in the rabies treatment centre of a major city hospital. First-aid measures should be started immediately (see Post-exposure prophylaxis, below).

Travellers should avoid contact with free-roaming animals, especially dogs and cats, and with wild and captive animals. For travellers who participate in caving/spelunking, casual exposure to cave air is not a concern, but cavers should be warned not to handle bats.

Vaccine

Vaccination against rabies is used in two distinct situations:

– to protect those who are at risk of exposure to rabies, i.e. pre-exposure vaccination;
– to prevent clinical rabies occurrence after exposure has occurred, usually following the bite of an animal suspected of having rabies, i.e. post-exposure prophylaxis.

The vaccines used for pre-exposure and post-exposure vaccination are the same, but the immunization schedule differs according to the type of application. Rabies immunoglobulin is used only for post-exposure prophylaxis. Modern vaccines of cell-culture or embryonated egg origin are safer and more effective than the older vaccines, which were produced in brain tissue. These modern rabies vaccines are now available in major urban centres of most countries of the developing world. Rabies immunoglobulin, on the other hand, is in short supply worldwide and may not be available even in major urban centres in many dog rabies-infected countries.

Pre-exposure vaccination

Pre-exposure vaccination should be offered to people at high risk of exposure to rabies, such as laboratory staff working with rabies virus, veterinarians, animal handlers and wildlife officers, and other individuals living in or travelling to areas where rabies is endemic. Travellers with extensive outdoor exposure in rural areas – such as might occur while running, bicycling, hiking, camping, backpacking, etc. – may be at risk, even if the duration of travel is short. Pre-exposure vaccination is advisable for children living in or visiting rabies-endemic areas, where they provide an easy target for rabid animals. Pre-exposure vaccination is also recommended for persons travelling to isolated areas or to areas where immediate access to appropriate medical care is limited or to countries where biologicals are in short supply and locally available rabies vaccines might be unsafe and/or ineffective.

Pre-exposure vaccination consists of three full intramuscular doses of cell-culture or embryonated egg origin rabies vaccine given on days 0, 7 and 21 or 28 (a few days' variation in the timing is not important). For adults, the vaccine should always be administered in the deltoid area of the arm; for young children (under 2 years of age), the anterolateral area of the thigh is recommended. Rabies vaccine should never be administered in the gluteal area: administration in this manner will result in lower neutralizing antibody titres.

To reduce the cost of cell-derived vaccines for pre-exposure rabies prophylaxis, intradermal vaccination in 0.1-ml volumes on days 0, 7 and either 21 or 28 may be considered. This method of administration is an acceptable alternative to the standard intramuscular administration, but it is technically more demanding and requires appropriate staff training and qualified medical supervision. As an open vial should not be kept for more than 6 hours, wastage can be avoided by vaccinating several people during that period. Concurrent use of chloroquine can reduce the antibody response to intradermal application of cell-culture rabies vaccines. People who are currently receiving malaria prophylaxis or who are unable to complete the entire three-dose pre-exposure series before starting malarial prophylaxis should therefore receive pre-exposure vaccination by the intramuscular route.

Rabies vaccines will induce long-lasting memory cells, giving rise to an accelerated immune response when a booster dose of vaccine is administered. Periodic booster injections are therefore not recommended for general travellers. However, in the event of exposure through the bite or scratch of an animal known or suspected to be rabid, persons who have previously received a complete series of pre- or post-exposure rabies vaccine (with cell-culture or embryonated egg vaccine) should receive two booster doses of vaccine. Ideally, the first dose should be administered on the day of exposure and the second 3 days later. This should be combined with thorough wound treatment (see Post-exposure prophylaxis, below). Rabies immunoglobulin is not required for previously vaccinated patients (as mentioned above).

Periodic booster injections are recommended only for people whose occupations put them at continuous or frequent risk of rabies exposure, e.g. rabies researchers, staff in diagnostic laboratories where rabies virus is present. For more information on continuous or frequent risk, see *WHO Expert Consultation on Rabies*.[1] For persons at continuous or frequent risk of rabies exposure who have previously received pre-exposure rabies vaccination, a booster vaccination consists of one dose of a cell-culture or embryonated egg rabies vaccine. In this case, a routine booster vaccination is administered if the serological titre of the person at risk falls below 0.5 IU/ml, the antibody level considered to be adequate.

Precautions and contraindications

Modern rabies vaccines are well tolerated. The frequency of minor adverse reactions (local pain, erythema, swelling and pruritus) varies widely from one report to another. Occasional systemic reactions (malaise, generalized aches and headaches) have been noted after both intramuscular and intradermal injections.

Type of vaccine:	Modern cell-culture or embryonated egg vaccine
Number of doses:	Three, one on each of days 0, 7 and 21 or 28, given i.m. (1 ml/dose) or i.d. (0.1 ml/per inoculation site)[a]
Booster:	Not routinely needed for general travellers[b]
Adverse reactions:	Minor local or systemic reactions

---

[1] *WHO Expert Consultation on Rabies: first report*. Geneva, World Health Organization, 2005 (WHO Technical Report Series, No. 931); available at www.who.int/rabies/Expert-ConsultationOnRabies.pdf

Before departure:	Pre-exposure prophylaxis for those planning a visit to a rabies-endemic country, especially if the visited area is far from major urban centres where appropriate care, including the availability of post-exposure rabies prophylaxis, is not assured.

[a] For information on which vaccines are recommended for intradermal use, see: http://www.who.int/rabies/human/postexp/en/index.html

[b] In the event of exposure through the bite or scratch of an animal known or suspected to be rabid, persons who have previously received a complete series of pre-exposure or post-exposure cell-culture or embryonated egg rabies vaccine should receive two booster doses of vaccine, the first dose ideally on the day of exposure and the second 3 days later. Rabies immunoglobulin should not be administered.

Rabies post-exposure prophylaxis

In a rabies-endemic area, the circumstances of an animal bite or other contact with an animal suspected to be rabid may require post-exposure prophylaxis. In such situations, medical advice should be obtained immediately.

Post-exposure prophylaxis to prevent the establishment of rabies infection involves first-aid treatment of the wound followed by administration of rabies vaccine; in the case of category III exposure, rabies immunoglobulin should also be administered.

Strict adherence to the WHO-recommended guidelines for optimal post-exposure rabies prophylaxis virtually guarantees protection from the disease. The administration of vaccine, and immunoglobulin if required, must be conducted by, or under the direct supervision of, a physician.

Post-exposure prophylaxis depends on the type of contact with the confirmed or suspect rabid animal, as follows:

Type of contact, exposure and recommended post-exposure prophylaxis

Category	Type of contact with a suspect or confirmed rabid domestic or wild[a] animal, or animal unavailable for testing	Type of exposure	Recommended post-exposure prophylaxis
I	Touching or feeding of animals Licks on intact skin	None	None, if reliable case history is available
II	Nibbling of uncovered skin Minor scratches or abrasions without bleeding	Minor	Administer vaccine immediately.[b] Stop treatment if animal remains healthy throughout an obser-

			vation period of 10 days[c] or is proved to be negative for rabies by a reliable laboratory using appropriate diagnostic techniques
III	Single or multiple transdermal bites or scratches, licks on broken skin Contamination of mucous membrane with saliva (i.e. licks) Exposures to bats[d]	Severe	Administer rabies immuno-globulin and vaccine immediately. Stop treatment if animal remains healthy throughout an observation period of 10 days or is found to be negative for rabies by a reliable laboratory using appro priate diagnostic techniques

[a] Exposure to rodents, rabbits and hares seldom, if ever, requires specific anti-rabies post-exposure prophylaxis.

[b] If an apparently healthy dog or cat in or from a low-risk area is placed under observation, the situation may warrant delaying initiation of treatment.

[c] This observation period applies only to dogs and cats. Except in the case of threatened or endangered species, other domestic and wild animals suspected to be rabid should be humanely killed and their tissues examined for the presence of rabies antigen using appropriate laboratory techniques.

[d] Post-exposure prophylaxis should be considered when contact between a human and a bat has occurred unless the exposed person can rule out a bite or scratch or exposure to a mucous membrane.

(1) Local treatment of wounds (first aid treatment)

Elimination of the rabies virus at the site of bite or scratch by chemical or physical means is an effective mechanism to aid in the protection against infection. Immediate washing and flushing for a minimum of 15 minutes with soap or detergent and water, or water alone, is imperative. Following washing, ethanol (70%) or iodine or povidone iodine should be applied. Most severe bite wounds are best treated by daily dressing. Suturing should be avoided; if it cannot be avoided, the wound should first be infiltrated with passive rabies immunization products and suturing delayed for several hours. This will allow diffusion of the antibody through the tissues before suturing is performed. Antibiotics and tetanus prophylaxis should be administered as appropriate for other wounds.

(2) Rabies biologicals for passive immunization:

Rabies immunoglobulins (RIG) should be administered in all category III exposures (as well as in category II exposures when the patient is immunosuppressed). Human rabies immunglobulin (HRIG) is mainly available in industrialized countries; both purified equine rabies immunoglobulin (ERIG) and human immunoglobulin are used in developing countries. F(ab')2 products have recently been developed from equine immunoglobulins. Given that the clearance of F(ab')2 fragments is more rapid than that of intact immunoglobulins, in case of multiple severe exposures, HRIG should preferably be used for passive immunization.

Dosage and administration: The dose for HRIG is 20 IU/kg body weight, and for ERIG and F(ab')2 products 40 IU/kg body weight. The full dose of rabies immunoglobulin, or as much as is anatomically feasible, should be administered into and around the wound site. Any remainder should be injected i.m. at a site distant from the site of vaccine administration. Multiple needle injections into the wound should be avoided. If the dose of rabies immunoglobulin is too small to infiltrate all wounds, as might be true of a severely bitten individual, the correct dosage of rabies immunoglobulin can be diluted in physiological buffered saline to ensure greater wound coverage.

HRIG gives rise to virtually no serious adverse reactions. ERIG is now highly purified and the occurrence of adverse events has been significantly reduced (<1–2%, compared with 40% for the original unpurified rabies antisera). F(ab')2 products were originally developed from equine immunoglobulins in order to reduce the severe adverse reactions initially described in association with the use of heterologous immunoglobulin products. Thus, they cause virtually no serious adverse reactions. Pregnancy, infancy, old age and concurrent illness are not contraindications for rabies post-exposure prophylaxis in the event of an exposure.

Rabies biologicals for passive immunization should not be administered later than 7 days after post-exposure vaccination with cell-culture or embryonated egg rabies vaccine has been initiated.

(3) Active immunization for post-exposure prophylaxis:

Highly purified and potent modern cell-culture or embryonated egg vaccines should be used. Cell-culture and embryonated egg vaccines can be administered either i.m. or i.d.

Intramuscular regimens: Two i.m. regimens are recommended for post-exposure vaccination; the five-dose regimen (Essen regimen) is the more commonly used:

- *Essen regimen*: this five-dose regimen is administered on days 0, 3, 7, 14 and 28 in the deltoid muscle.

- *Zagreb or '2-1-1' regimen*: administered as 2 doses on day 0 (one dose in the right and one in the left deltoid), and one dose on each of days 7 and 21 in the deltoid muscle.

Intradermal regimens: Intradermal administration of cell-culture and embryonated egg rabies vaccines has been successfully used in many developing countries that cannot afford the five-dose intramuscular schedule. Intradermal schedules have been evaluated and used extensively for post-exposure prophylaxis in some developing countries to replace nerve–tissue vaccines where intramuscular vaccination regimens are not an alternative from an economic viewpoint. Intradermal injections should be administered by staff well trained in the technique.

WHO recommends the following intradermal regimens and vaccines for use by the intradermal route:

- *8-site intradermal method (8-0-4-0-1-1)*: one intradermal injection at 8 sites on day 0 (one in each upper arm, one in each lateral thigh, one on each side of the suprascapular region, and one on each side of the lower quadrant region of the abdomen); one injection at 4 sites on day 7 (one in each upper arm and in lateral thigh); and one injection at one site on days 30 and 90 (one upper arm).

For use with: human diploid cell vaccine (HDCV) (Imovax™) and purified chick embryo cell vaccine (PCECV) (Rabipur™). Both vaccines at 0.1 ml per intradermal site.

- *2-site intradermal method (2-2-2-0-2)*: one intradermal injection at 2 sites on days 0, 3, 7 and 28.

For use with: 0.1 ml for purified vero cell rabies vaccine (PVRV) (Verorab™); 0.1 ml for PCECV (Rabipur™).

Post-exposure rabies prophylaxis	
1.	**Wound treatment:** Thorough washing of the wound with soap/detergent and water, followed by the application of ethanol or an aqueous solution of iodine or povidone.
2.	**Passive immunization:** Human rabies immunglobulin or equine rabies immunglobulin or F(ab')2 products for category III exposure (see table, above). Human rabies immunoglobulin should be used in case of multiple severe exposure. Passive immunization should be administered just before administration of the first dose of vaccine given in the post-exposure prophylaxis regimen. If it is not immediately available, passive immunization can be administered up until the seventh day after the primary series of post-exposure prophylaxis (with cell-culture or embryonated egg rabies vaccine) was initiated.
3.	**Active immunization:** Cell-culture or embryonated egg rabies vaccines should always be used for post-exposure prophylaxis (see regimens above).[a]

Post-exposure prophylaxis in previously vaccinated individuals: For persons who have previously received a full course of cell-culture or embryonated egg rabies vaccine, post-exposure prophylaxis consists of a series of two booster doses of vaccine given either intramuscularly or intradermally on days 0 and 3. It is not necessary to administer passive immunization products.

ᵃ Post-exposure prophylaxis can be stopped if the suspect animal is proved by appropriate laboratory examination to be free of rabies or, in the case of domestic dogs and cats, if the animal remains healthy throughout a 10-day observation period.

TICK-BORNE ENCEPHALITIS

Disease and occurrence

See Chapter 5.

Risk for travellers

Travellers who walk and camp in infested areas during the tick season (usually spring to early autumn) are at risk and should be vaccinated. Some degree of protection is afforded by clothing that covers as much skin as possible and by applying insect repellent.

Vaccine

The vaccine should be offered only to high-risk travellers. Two vaccines are available in Europe, in adult and paediatric formulations. These are inactivated whole-cell vaccines containing a suspension of purified tick-borne encephalitis virus grown on chick embryo cells and inactivated with formaldehyde. Both provide safe and reliable protection. Immunity is induced against all variants of the tick-borne encephalitis virus including the European and Far Eastern subtypes. Two doses of 0.5 ml should be given i.m. 4–12 weeks apart. A third dose is given 9–12 months after the second dose and confers immunity for 3 years. Booster doses are required to maintain immunity and should be given every 3 years if the risk continues. Outside endemic countries, the vaccines may not be licensed and will have to be obtained by special request.

Precautions and contraindications

Occasional local reactions may occur, such as reddening and swelling around the injection site, swelling of the regional lymph nodes or general reactions (e.g. fatigue, pain in the limb, nausea and headache). Rarely, there may be fever above 38 °C for a short time, vomiting or transient rash. In very rare cases, neuritis of varying severity may be seen, although the etiological relationship to vaccination is uncertain.

The vaccination has been suspected of aggravating autoimmune diseases such as multiple sclerosis and iridocyclitis, but this remains unproven. Hypersensitivity to thiomersal (a vaccine preservative) is a contraindication.

Type of vaccine:	Killed
Number of doses:	Two, given i.m. 4–12 weeks apart, plus booster
Booster:	9–12 months after second dose
Contraindications:	Hypersensitivity to the vaccine preservative thiomersal; adverse reaction to previous dose
Adverse reactions:	Local reactions occasionally; rarely fever
Before departure:	Second dose 2 weeks before departure
Recommended for:	High-risk individuals only
Special precautions:	Avoid ticks; remove ticks immediately if bitten

TYPHOID FEVER

Disease and occurrence

See Chapter 5.

Risk for travellers

All travellers to endemic areas are at potential risk of typhoid fever, although the risk is generally low in tourist and business centres where standards of accommodation, sanitation and food hygiene are high. The risk is particularly high in the Indian subcontinent. Even vaccinated individuals should take care to avoid consumption of potentially contaminated food and water as the vaccine does not confer 100% protection.

Vaccine

Travellers to countries where the risk of typhoid fever is high, especially those staying for longer than a month, those exposed to conditions of poor hygiene, and those visiting the Indian subcontinent and destinations where there is the possibility of antibiotic-resistant organisms, may be offered one of the following vaccines.

- Oral Ty21a. This live, attenuated mutant strain of Salmonella typhi Ty21a, supplied as enteric coated capsules, is given orally in three doses (four in North America) 2 days apart, and produces protection 7 days after the final dose. Seven years after the final dose the protective efficacy is 67% in residents of endemic areas but may be less for travellers. A liquid formulation is no longer available.

– Injectable Vi CPS. Capsular Vi polysaccharide vaccine (Vi CPS), containing 25 µg of polysaccharide per dose, is given i.m. in a single dose and produces protection 7 days after injection. In endemic areas, the protective efficacy is 72% after 1.5 years and 50% 3 years after vaccination.

Both vaccines are safe and effective, currently licensed and available and should now replace the previous, more reactogenic, inactivated whole-cell typhoid vaccine. However, their efficacy in children under 2 years of age has not been demonstrated.

A combined typhoid/hepatitis A vaccine is also available in some countries.

Precautions and contraindications

Proguanil, mefloquine and antibiotics should be stopped from 3 days before until 3 days after giving Ty21a.

Comparison of the adverse effects of typhoid vaccines shows that more systemic reactions (e.g. fever) occur after i.m. administration of inactivated vaccine than after either Ty21a or Vi CPS. No serious adverse effects have been reported following administration of Ty 21a or Vi CPS.

These vaccines are not recommended for use in infant immunization programmes: there is insufficient information on their efficacy in children under 2 years of age.

Type of vaccine:	Oral Ty21a and injectable Vi CPS
Number of doses:	One of Vi CPS, i.m. Three or four of live Ty21a, given orally at 2-day intervals as enteric coated capsule
Booster:	Every 2 to 3 years for Vi CPS; for Ty21a see package insert[a]
Contraindications:	Proguanil, mefloquine and antibiotics 3 days before or after starting Ty21a
Adverse reactions:	None significant
Before departure:	1 week
Recommended for:	Travellers to high-risk areas and travellers staying longer than 1 month or likely to consume food or beverages away from the usual tourist routes in developing countries

Special precautions: Vi CPS – not under 2 years of age; avoid proguanil, mefloquine and antibiotics with Ty21a

[a] The duration of protection following Ty21a immunization is not well defined and may vary with vaccine dose and possibly with subsequent exposures to Salmonella typhi (natural booster). In Australia and Europe, 3 tablets are given on days 1, 3, and 5; this series is repeated every year for persons travelling from non-endemic to endemic countries, and every 3 years for persons living in endemic areas. In North America, 4 tablets are given on days 1, 3, 5, and 7 and revaccination is recommended only after 5 years (USA) or 7 years (Canada) for all, regardless of typhoid fever endemicity in the country of residence.

YELLOW FEVER

Disease and occurrence

See Chapter 5.

Risk for travellers

The normally low risk to travellers increases with travel to jungle areas in endemic countries and in or near cities during urban outbreaks. Areas where yellow fever virus is present far exceed those officially reported. The risk of exposure to infection can be reduced by taking measures to prevent mosquito bites (see Chapter 3). It should be noted that the mosquito vectors of yellow fever bite mostly during daylight hours. Although reported cases of human disease are the principal indicator of disease risk, some countries may have no reported cases, either because of a high level of vaccine coverage against yellow fever in the population or because poor surveillance resulted in no cases being reported. However, the risk of yellow fever may still persist as the virus, the vector or the animal reservoir is still present.

Vaccine

The 17D vaccine, which is based on a live, attenuated viral strain, is the only commercially available yellow fever vaccine. It is given as a single subcutaneous (or intramuscular) injection. Yellow fever vaccine is highly effective (approaching 100%), while the disease may be fatal in adults who are not immune. With few exceptions (see below), vaccination is recommended for all travellers to countries or areas where there is a risk of yellow fever transmission (see country list and Annex 1).

Precautions and contraindications

Tolerance of the vaccine is generally excellent – only 2–5% of vaccine recipients have mild reactions, including myalgia and headache. Contraindications include true allergy to egg protein, cellular immunodeficiency (congenital or acquired, the latter sometimes being only temporary) and symptomatic HIV infection. Many industrialized countries administer yellow fever vaccine to persons with symptomatic HIV infection provided that the CD4 count is at least 200 cells/mm^3. Asymptomatic HIV-positive individuals may have a reduced response to the vaccine. There is a theoretical risk of harm to the fetus if the vaccine is given during pregnancy, but this must be weighed against the risk to the mother of remaining unvaccinated and travelling to a high-risk zone. (However, pregnant women should be advised not to travel to areas where exposure to yellow fever may occur.) Encephalitis has been reported as a rare event following vaccination of infants under 9 months of age; as a result, the vaccine is contraindicated in children aged under 6 months and is not recommended for those aged 6–8 months.

There have been recent reports of a small number of cases of serious viscerotropic disease, including deaths, following yellow fever vaccination; most of these reactions occurred in elderly persons. The risk of yellow fever vaccine-associated viscerotropic disease appears to be limited to the first immunization. The frequency of such reactions remains uncertain, although estimates based on Brazilian experience (including routine childhood immunization) indicate a risk in the order of 1 per 10 million doses. Comparative risk estimates from the USA (mainly protection of adult travellers) are 1 per 200 000–300 000 doses and 1 per 40 000–50 000 doses for vaccinees over 60 years of age. A history of thymus disease has been identified as one of the risk factors.

The risk to unvaccinated individuals who visit countries where there may be yellow fever transmission is far greater than the risk of a vaccine-related adverse event, and it remains important for all travellers at risk to be vaccinated. Nonetheless, yellow fever vaccination should not be prescribed for individuals who are not at risk of exposure to infection. Yellow fever vaccination should be encouraged as a key prevention strategy, but it is important to screen travel itineraries, particularly of older travellers, and carefully evaluate the potential risk of systemic illness after yellow fever vaccination.

Type of vaccine:	Live, attenuated
Number of doses:	One priming dose of 0.5 ml
Booster:	10-yearly (if re-certification is needed)
Contraindications:	Egg allergy; immunodeficiency from medication, disease or symptomatic HIV infection; hypersensitivity to a previous dose; pregnancy (see text above)
Adverse reactions:	Rarely, encephalitis or hepatic failure

Before departure:	International certificate of vaccination becomes valid 10 days after vaccination
Recommended for:	All travellers to endemic zones and wherever mandatory
Special precautions:	Not for infants under 9 months of age; restrictions in pregnancy

Mandatory vaccination

Yellow fever

Mandatory vaccination against yellow fever is carried out to prevent the importation of yellow fever virus into vulnerable countries. These are countries where yellow fever does not occur but where the mosquito vector and non-human primate hosts are present. Importation of the virus by an infected traveller could potentially lead to the establishment of infection in mosquitoes and primates, with a consequent risk of infection for the local population. In such cases, vaccination is an entry requirement for all travellers arriving from countries, including airport transit, where there is a risk of yellow fever transmission.

If yellow fever vaccination is contraindicated for medical reasons, a medical certificate is required for exemption.

The international yellow fever vaccination certificate becomes valid 10 days after vaccination and remains valid for a period of 10 years.

For information on countries that require proof of yellow fever vaccination as a condition of entry, see country list.

Travellers should be aware that the absence of a requirement for vaccination does not imply that there is no risk of exposure to yellow fever in the country.

The international certificate of vaccination is reproduced with explanatory notes at the end of the chapter. A revision of the International Health Regulations was adopted on 23 May 2005 by the World Health Assembly and these Regulations will enter into force in June 2007 (see Annex 2). As from June 2007, the current "International certificate of vaccination or revaccination against yellow fever" will be replaced by the "International certificate of vaccination or prophylaxis". Clinicians who will issue the certificate should note that the main difference to the current certificate is that they have to specify in writing in the space provided that the disease for which the certificate is issued is "yellow fever".

Meningococcal disease

Vaccination against meningococcal disease is required by Saudi Arabia for pilgrims visiting Mecca for the Hajj (annual pilgrimage) or for the Umrah.

Following the occurrence of cases of meningococcal disease associated with *N. meningitidis* W-135 among pilgrims in 2000 and 2001, the current requirement is for vaccination with tetravalent vaccine (A, C, Y and W-135). Vaccine requirements for Hajj pilgrims are issued each year and published in the Weekly Epidemiological Record.

Poliomyelitis

Some polio-free countries may require travellers from endemic countries to be immunized against polio in order to obtain an entry visa. Updates are published in the *Weekly Epidemiological Record*. For more information on Hajj visa requirements, see Chapter 9.

Special groups

Infants and young children

Because not all vaccines can be administered to the very young, it is especially important to ensure protection against health hazards such as foodborne illnesses and mosquito bites by means other than vaccination. Some vaccines can be administered in the first few days of life (BCG, oral poliomyelitis vaccine, hepatitis B). Other vaccines cannot be given before a certain time, e.g. diphtheria/tetanus/pertussis, diphtheria/tetanus, inactivated poliomyelitis vaccine should not be given before 6 weeks of age, Japanese encephalitis not before 6 months and yellow fever not before 9 months of age. Because it may be difficult to reduce children's exposure to environmental dangers, it is particularly important to ensure that their routine vaccinations are fully up to date. A child who travels abroad before completing the full schedule of routine vaccines is at risk from vaccine-preventable diseases.

Adolescents and young adults

Adolescents and young adults make up the largest group of travellers and the group most likely to acquire sexually transmitted diseases or other travel-related infections. They are particularly at risk when travelling on a limited budget and using accommodation of poor standard (e.g. when backpacking), as well as from a lifestyle that may include risky sexual behaviour and other risks taken under the influence of alcohol or drugs. Because risk reduction through behaviour modification may not be reliable, this age group should be strongly encouraged to accept all appropriate vaccines before travel and to adhere to other precautions for avoiding infectious diseases.

Frequent travellers

Individuals who travel widely, usually by air, often become lax about taking precautions regarding their health. Having travelled numerous times without major health upsets, they may neglect to check that they are up to date with vaccination. Such travellers pose a special problem for health advisers who should, nonetheless, encourage compliance.

Pregnancy

Pregnancy should not deter a woman from receiving vaccines that are safe and will protect both her health and that of her unborn child. However, care must be taken to avoid the inappropriate administration of certain vaccines that could harm the unborn baby. Killed or inactivated vaccines, toxoids and polysaccharides can generally be given during pregnancy, as can oral polio vaccine. Live vaccines are generally contraindicated because of largely theoretical risks to the baby. Measles, mumps, rubella, BCG, varicella and yellow fever vaccines should therefore be avoided in pregnancy. The risks and benefits should nevertheless be examined in each individual case. Vaccination against yellow fever may be considered after the sixth month of pregnancy when the risk from exposure is deemed greater than the risk to the fetus (see Table 6.2). However, pregnant women should be advised not to travel to areas where there is a risk of exposure to yellow fever. For more detailed information, see the specific vaccine position papers at: http://www.who.int/immunization/documents/positionpapers_intro/en/index.html

Elderly travellers

Vaccination of healthy elderly travellers does not differ in principle from vaccination of younger adults. However, special considerations arise if the elderly traveller has not been fully immunized in the past and/or has existing medical problems.

Many elderly people may have never been vaccinated with the vaccines used in routine childhood immunization programmes, or may have neglected to keep up the recommended schedule of booster doses. As a consequence, they may be susceptible to diseases such as diphtheria, tetanus and poliomyelitis as well as to other infections present at the travel destination.

Table 6.2 **Vaccination in pregnancy**

Vaccine	Use in pregnancy	Comments
BCG[a]	No	
Cholera	Yes, administer oral inactivated vaccine if indicated	
Hepatitis A	Yes, administer if indicated	Safety not determined
Hepatitis B	Yes, administer if indicated	
Influenza	Yes, administer if indicated	In some circumstances – consult a physician
Japanese encephalitis		Safety not determined
Measles[a]	No	
Meningococcal disease	Yes, administer if indicated	
Mumps[a]	No	
Poliomyelitis OPV[a]	Yes, administer if indicated	
IPV	Yes, administer if indicated	Normally avoided
Rubella[a]	No	
Tetanus/diphtheria	Yes, administer if indicated	
Rabies	Yes, administer if indicated	
Typhoid Ty21a[a]	Safety not determined	
Varicella[a]	No	
Yellow fever[a]	Yes, administer if indicated	Avoid unless at high risk

[a] Live vaccine.

Elderly travellers who have never been vaccinated should be offered a full primary course of vaccination against diphtheria, tetanus, poliomyelitis and hepatitis B. In addition, those who are not immune to hepatitis A should be vaccinated against this disease before travelling to a developing country.

Since the elderly are at risk for severe and complicated influenza, regular annual vaccination is recommended. For travellers from one hemisphere to the other, vaccine against the currently circulating strains of influenza is unlikely to be obtainable before arrival at the travel destination. Those arriving shortly before, or early during, the influenza season, and planning to stay for more than 2–3 weeks, should arrange vaccination as soon as possible after arrival. Pneumococcal vaccine should also be considered for elderly travellers in view of the risk of pneumococcal pneumonia following influenza infection.

Special considerations arise in the case of elderly travellers with pre-existing chronic health problems (see below).

Travellers with chronic medical problems

Travellers with chronic medical conditions involving impaired immunity, including cancer, diabetes mellitus, HIV infection and treatment with immunosuppressive drugs, may be at risk of severe complications following administration of vaccines that contain live organisms. Consequently, it may be advisable to avoid measles, oral polio, yellow fever, varicella and BCG vaccines for these travellers. For travel to a country where yellow fever vaccination is mandatory, a medical certificate will be required to obtain exemption.

Travellers with chronic cardiovascular and/or respiratory conditions or diabetes mellitus are at high risk for severe influenza and its complications. Regular annual vaccination against influenza is recommended. For travel from one hemisphere to the other shortly before, or early, during the influenza season, vaccination should be sought as soon as possible after arrival at the travel destination.

For those who lack a functional spleen, additional vaccines are advised: Hib, meningococcal vaccine (conjugate C or quadrivalent conjugate vaccine) and pneumococcal vaccination should be considered, in addition to regular vaccination against influenza.

HIV-positive and immunocompromised travellers

The likelihood of successful immunization is reduced in some HIV-infected children and adults, but the risk of serious adverse effects remains low. Asymptomatic HIV-infected children should be immunized according to standard schedules. With certain exceptions, symptomatic HIV-positive individuals should also be immunized as usual. Both measles and oral poliomyelitis vaccines may be given to persons with symptomatic HIV infection, but special attention should be paid to measles vaccination. Some vaccinations are contraindicated for this group:

● Measles vaccine has generally been recommended for individuals with moderate immunodeficiency if there is even a low risk of contracting wild measles from the community. A low level of risk is associated with use of measles vaccine in individuals who are HIV-infected and whose immune system is impaired. Where the risk of contracting wild measles infection is negligible, it may be preferable to avoid use of the vaccine.

- Yellow fever vaccine is not recommended for symptomatic HIV-positive adults and children. It is not certain whether yellow fever vaccine poses a risk for asymptomatic HIV-infected persons. Any adverse reactions to the vaccine occurring in HIV-positive individuals should be reported to WHO. In many industrialized countries, yellow fever vaccine is administered to people with symptomatic HIV infection or suffering from other immunodeficiency diseases, provided that their CD4 count is at least 200 cells/mm^3 and if they plan to visit areas where epidemic or endemic yellow fever actually occurs.

- BCG vaccine should not be given to individuals with symptomatic HIV/AIDS.

Adverse reactions and contraindications

Reactions to vaccines

While vaccines are generally both effective and safe, no vaccine is totally safe for all recipients. Vaccination may sometimes cause certain mild side-effects: local reaction, slight fever and other systemic symptoms may develop as part of the normal immune response. In addition, certain components of the vaccine (e.g. aluminium adjuvant, antibiotics or preservatives) occasionally cause reactions. A successful vaccine reduces these reactions to a minimum while inducing maximum immunity. Serious reactions are rare. Health workers who administer vaccines have an obligation to inform recipients of known adverse reactions and the likelihood of their occurrence.

A known contraindication should be clearly marked on a traveller's vaccination card, so that the vaccine may be avoided in future. In exceptional circumstances, the medical adviser may consider the risk of a particular disease to be greater than the theoretical risk of administering the vaccine and will advise vaccination.

Common mild vaccine reactions

Most vaccines produce some mild local and/or systemic reactions relatively frequently. These reactions generally occur within a day or two of immunization. However, the systemic symptoms that may arise with measles or MMR vaccine occur 5–12 days after vaccination. Fever and/or rash occur in 5–15% of measles/MMR vaccine recipients during this time, but only 3% are attributable to the vaccine; the rest may be classed as background events, i.e. normal events of childhood.

Uncommon, severe adverse reactions

Most of the rare vaccine reactions (detailed in Table 6.3) are self-limiting and do not lead to long-term problems. Anaphylaxis, for example, although potentially fatal, can be treated and has no long-term effects.

All serious reactions should be reported immediately to the relevant national health authority and marked on the vaccination card. In addition, the patient and relatives should be instructed to avoid the vaccination in the future.

Table 6.3 **Uncommon severe adverse reactions**

Vaccine	Possible adverse reaction per million doses	Expected rate[a]
BCG	Suppurative lymphadenitis	100–1 000 (mostly in immunodeficient individuals)
	BCG-osteitis	1–700 (rarely with current vaccines)
	Disseminated BCG infection	0.19–1.56
Cholera	NR[b]	—
DTP	Persistent crying	1 000–60 000
	Seizures	570
	Hypotonic–hyporesponsive episode	570
	Anaphylaxis	20
Haemophilus influenzae	NR	—
Hepatitis A	NR	—
Hepatitis B[c]	Anaphylaxis	1–2
Influenza	Guillain–Barré syndrome	<1
Japanese encephalitis	Mouse-brain only – neurological event	Rare
	Hypersensitivity	1 800–6 400
Measles	Febrile seizure	333
	Thrombocytopenic purpura	33–45
	Anaphylaxis	1–50
	Encephalitis	1 (unproven)
Meningococcal disease	Anaphylaxis	1
Mumps	Depends on strain – aseptic meningitis	0–500
Pneumococcal	Anaphylaxis	Very rare

Vaccine	Possible adverse reaction per million doses	Expected rate[a]
Poliomyelitis (OPV)	Vaccine-associated paralytic poliomyelitis	1.4–3.4
Poliomyelitis (IPV)	NR	—
Rabies	Animal brain tissue only – neuroparalysis	17–44
	Cell-derived – allergic reactions	Rare
Rubella	Arthralgia/arthritis/arthropathy	None or very rare
Tetanus	Brachial neuritis	5–10
	Anaphylaxis	1–6
Tick-borne encephalitis	NR	—
Typhoid fever	Parenteral vaccine – various	Very rare
	Oral vaccine – NR	—
Yellow fever	Encephalitis (<6 months)	500–4 000
	Allergy/anaphylaxis	5–20
	Viscerotropic disease	0.04–3
		20 for vaccinees above 60 years of age

[a] Precise rate may vary with survey method.

[b] NR = none reported.

[c] Although there have been anecdotal reports of demyelinating disease following hepatitis B vaccine, there is no scientific evidence for a causal relationship.

Contraindications

The main contraindications to the administration of vaccines are summarized in Table 6.4.

Table 6.4 **Contraindications to vaccines**

Vaccine	Contraindications
All	An anaphylactic reaction[a] following a previous dose of a particular vaccine is a true contraindication to further immunization with the antigen concerned and a subsequent dose should not be given. Current serious illness
MMR, BCG, live JE, varicella	Pregnancy Severe immunodeficiency
Yellow fever	Severe egg allergy Severe immunodeficiency (from medication, disease or symptomatic) Pregnancy HIV infection[b]
BCG	HIV infection
Influenza	Severe egg allergy
Pertussis-containing vaccines	Anaphylactic reaction to a previous dose Delay vaccination in case of evolving neurological disease (e.g. uncontrolled epilepsy or progressive encephalopathy).

[a] Generalized urticaria, difficulty in breathing, swelling of the mouth and throat, hypotension or shock.

[b] In many industrialized countries, yellow fever vaccine is administered to individuals with symptomatic HIV infection or who are suffering from other immunodeficiency diseases, provided that their CD4 count is at least 200 cells/mm3 and if they plan to visit areas where epidemic or endemic yellow fever actually occurs.

Further reading

Global Influenza Surveillance Network (FluNet): http://www.who.int/GlobalAtlas/

Information on safety of vaccines from the Global Advisory Committee on Vaccine Safety: http://www.who.int/vaccine_safety/en/

WHO information on vaccine preventable diseases: http://www.who.int/immunization/en/

WHO vaccine position papers: http://www.who.int/immunization/documents/positionpapers_intro/en/index.html

International certificate of vaccination

The certificate must be *printed* in English and French; an additional language may be added. It must be *completed* in English or French; an additional language may be used.

The international certificate of vaccination is an *individual* certificate. It should not be used collectively. Separate certificates should be issued for children; the information should not be incorporated in the mother's certificate.

An international certificate is valid only if the yellow fever vaccine used has been approved by WHO and if the vaccinating centre has been designated by the national health administration for the area in which the centre is situated. The date should be recorded in the following sequence: day, month, year, with the month written in letters, e.g. 8 January 2007.

A certificate issued to a child who is unable to write should be signed by a parent or guardian. For illiterates, the signature should be indicated by their mark certified by another person.

Although a nurse may carry out the vaccination under the direct supervision of a qualified medical practitioner, the certificate must be signed by the person authorized by the national health administration. The official stamp of the centre is not an accepted substitute for a personal signature.

> Signature of person vaccinated
> Signature de la personne vaccinée

> e.g.: 8 January 2007
> ex.: 8 janvier 2007

> Signature required
> (rubber stamp not accepted)
> Signature exigée (le cachet
> n'est pas suffisant)

> Official stamp
> Cachet officiel

WHO 881091

International certificate of vaccination or revaccination against yellow fever
Certificat international de vaccination ou de revaccination contre la fièvre jaune

is is to certify that :oussigné(e) certifie que	Ole OLSEN	date of birth né(e) le	8 Nov. 1945	sex sexe	M

ose signature follows int la signature suit — *C. Olsen*

on the date indicated been vaccinated or revaccinated against yellow fever.
é vacciné(e) ou revacciné(e) contre la fièvre jaune à la date indiquée.

Date	Signature and professional status of vaccinator Signature et titre du vaccinateur	Manufacturer and batch no. of vaccine Fabricant du vaccin et numéro du lot	Official stamp of vaccinating centre Cachet officiel du centre de vaccination
8 January 2007	Dr John Doe M.D.	R.I.V. 63007	

This certificate is valid only if the vaccine used has been approved by the World Health Organization and if the vaccinating centre has been designated by the health administration for the territory in which that centre is situated.

The validity of this certificate shall extend for a period of 10 years, beginning 10 days after the date of vaccination or, in the event of a revaccination within such period of 10 years, from the date of that revaccination.

This certificate must be signed in his own hand by a medical practitioner or other person authorized by the national health administration; an official stamp is not an accepted substitute for a signature.

Any amendment of this certificate, or erasure, or failure to complete any part of it, may render it invalid.

Ce certificat n'est valable que si le vaccin employé a été approuvé par l'Organisation mondiale de la Santé et si le centre de vaccination a été habilité par l'administration sanitaire du territoire dans lequel ce centre est situé.

La validité de ce certificat couvre une période de 10 ans commençant 10 jours après la date de la vaccination ou, dans le cas d'une revaccination au cours de cette période de 10 ans, le jour de cette revaccination.

Ce certificat doit être signé de sa propre main par un médecin ou une autre personne habilitée par l'administration sanitaire nationale, un cachet officiel ne pouvant être considéré comme tenant lieu de signature.

Toute correction ou rature sur le certificat ou l'omission d'une quelconque des mentions qu'il comporte peut affecter sa validité.

International certificate of vaccination or prophylaxis

A revision of the International Health Regulations, referred to as IHR (2005), was unanimously adopted on 23 May 2005 by the World Health Assembly and these Regulations will enter into force in June 2007 (see Annex 2). As from 15 June 2007, the current "International certificate of vaccination or revaccination against yellow fever" will be replaced by the "International certificate of vaccination or prophylaxis", as follows:

Model international certificate of vaccination or prophylaxis

This is to certify that [name] ...., date of birth ....,

sex ....,

nationality ...., national identification document, if applicable

......................................,

whose signature follows ....

has on the date indicated been vaccinated or received prophylaxis against [name of disease or condition] in accordance with the International Health Regulations.

Vaccine or pro- phylaxis	Date	Signature and professional status of supervising clinician	Manufacturer and batch no. of vaccine or prophylaxis	Certificate valid from .... until	Official stamp of administering centre
1.					
2.					

This certificate is valid only if the vaccine or prophylaxis used has been approved by the World Health Organization.[1]

---

[1] See http://www.who.int/immunization_standards/vaccine_quality/pq_suppliers/en/index. html WHO Technical Report Series, No. 872, 1998, Annex 1 (www.who.int/biologicals). *Note*: since this list was issued, the following changes have taken place: Evans Medical is now Novartis Vaccines; Connaught Laboratories and Pasteur Merieux are now sanofi pasteur; Robert Koch Institute has ceased production.

This certificate must be signed in the hand of the clinician, who shall be a medical practitioner or other authorized health worker, supervising the administration of the vaccine or prophylaxis. The certificate must also bear the official stamp of the administering centre; however, this shall not be an accepted substitute for the signature.

Any amendment of this certificate, or erasure, or failure to complete any part of it, may render it invalid.

The validity of this certificate shall extend until the date indicated for the particular vaccination or prophylaxis. The certificate shall be fully completed in English or in French. The certificate may also be completed in another language on the same document, in addition to either English or French.

CHAPTER 7

Malaria

General considerations

Malaria is a common and life-threatening disease in many tropical and subtropical areas. It is currently endemic in over 100 countries, which are visited by more than 125 million international travellers every year.

Each year many international travellers fall ill with malaria while visiting countries where the disease is endemic, and well over 10 000 are reported to fall ill after returning home. Due to under-reporting, the real figure may be as high as 30 000. International travellers from non-endemic areas are at high risk of malaria and its consequences because they lack immunity. Immigrants from endemic areas who now live in non-endemic areas and return to their home countries to visit friends and relatives are similarly at risk because of waning or absent immunity. Fever occurring in a traveller within three months of leaving a malaria-endemic area is a medical emergency and should be investigated urgently.

Travellers who fall ill during travel may find it difficult to access reliable medical care. Travellers who develop malaria upon return to a non-endemic country present particular problems: doctors may be unfamiliar with malaria, the diagnosis may be delayed, and effective antimalarial medicines may not be registered and/or available, resulting in high case-fatality rates.

Cause

Human malaria is caused by four different species of the protozoan parasite *Plasmodium: Plasmodium falciparum, P. vivax, P. ovale* and *P. malariae.*

Transmission

The malaria parasite is transmitted by female *Anopheles* mosquitoes, which bite mainly between sunset and sunrise.

Nature of the disease

Malaria is an acute febrile illness with an incubation period of 7 days or longer. Thus, a febrile illness developing less than one week after the first possible exposure is not malaria.

The most severe form is caused by *P. falciparum*, in which variable clinical features include fever, chills, headache, muscular aching and weakness, vomiting, cough, diarrhoea and abdominal pain; other symptoms related to organ failure may supervene, such as acute renal failure, generalized convulsions, circulatory collapse, followed by coma and death. In endemic areas it is estimated that about 1% of patients with *P. falciparum* infection die of the disease; mortality in non-immune travellers with untreated falciparum infection is significantly higher. The initial symptoms, which may be mild, may not be easy to recognize as being due to malaria. It is important that the possibility of falciparum malaria is considered in all cases of unexplained fever starting at any time between 7 days after the first possible exposure to malaria and 3 months (or, rarely, later) after the last possible exposure. Any individual who experiences a fever in this interval should immediately seek diagnosis and effective treatment, and inform medical personnel of the possible exposure to malaria infection. Falciparum malaria may be fatal if treatment is delayed beyond 24 hours.

Young children, pregnant women, people living with HIV/AIDS and elderly travellers are particularly at risk. Malaria in non-immune pregnant travellers increases the risk of maternal death, miscarriage, stillbirth and neonatal death.

The forms of malaria caused by other *Plasmodium* species cause significant morbidity but are rarely life-threatening. *P. vivax* and *P. ovale* can remain dormant in the liver. Relapses caused by these persistent liver forms ("hypnozoites") may appear months, and rarely up to 2 years, after exposure. They are not prevented by current chemoprophylactic regimens, with the exception of primaquine. Latent blood infection with *P. malariae* may be present for many years, but it is not life-threatening.

Chemoprophylaxis and treatment of falciparum malaria are becoming more complex because *P. falciparum* is increasingly resistant to various antimalarial drugs. Chloroquine resistance of *P. vivax* is rare and was first reported in the late 1980s in Indonesia and Papua New Guinea. Focal "true" chloroquine resistance (i.e. in patients with adequate blood levels at day of failure) or prophylactic and/or treatment failure have since also been observed in Brazil, Colombia, Ethiopia, Guyana, India, Myanmar, Peru, the Republic of Korea, Solomon Islands, Thailand and Turkey. Chloroquine-resistant *P. malariae* has been reported from Indonesia.

Geographical distribution

The current distribution of malaria in the world is shown in the map on page 88. Affected countries and territories are listed at the end of this chapter, as well as in the Country list. The risk for travellers of contracting malaria is highly variable from country to country and even between areas in a country, and this must be considered in any discussion of appropriate preventive measures.

In many endemic countries, the main urban areas – but not necessarily the outskirts of towns – are free of malaria transmission. However, malaria can occur in the main urban areas of Africa and, to a lesser extent, India. There is usually less risk at altitudes above 1500 metres but, in favourable climatic conditions, the disease can occur at altitudes up to almost 3000 metres. The risk of infection may also vary according to the season, being highest at the end of the rainy season or soon after.

There is no risk of malaria in many tourist destinations in South-East Asia, Latin America and the Caribbean.

Risk for travellers

During the transmission season in malaria-endemic areas, all non-immune travellers exposed to mosquito bites, especially between dusk and dawn, are at risk of malaria. This includes previously semi-immune travellers who have lost or partially lost their immunity during stays of 6 months or more in non-endemic areas. Children of people who have migrated to non-endemic areas are particularly at risk when they return to malarious areas to visit friends and relatives.

Culturally sensitive approaches are needed to advise different groups at risk. Most cases of falciparum malaria in travellers occur because of poor adherence to, or complete failure to use, prophylactic drug regimens, or use of inappropriate medicines, combined with failure to take adequate precautions against mosquito bites. Late-onset vivax and ovale malaria may occur despite effective prophylaxis. Studies on travellers' behaviour have shown that adherence can be improved if travellers are informed of the risk of infection and believe in the benefit of prevention strategies.

Travellers to countries where the degree of malaria transmission varies in different areas should seek advice on the risk in the specific zones that they will be visiting. If specific information is not available before travelling, it is recommended that precautions appropriate for the highest reported risk for the area or country should be taken; these precautions can be adjusted when more information becomes available on arrival. This applies particularly to individuals backpacking to remote places and visiting areas where diagnostic facilities and medical care are not readily available. Travellers staying overnight in rural areas may be at highest risk.

Precautions

Travellers and their advisers should note the four principles – the ABCD – of malaria protection:

- Be **A**ware of the risk, the incubation period, and the main symptoms.
- Avoid being **B**itten by mosquitoes, especially between dusk and dawn.
- Take antimalarial drugs (**C**hemoprophylaxis) when appropriate, to prevent infection from developing into clinical disease.
- Immediately seek **D**iagnosis and treatment if a fever develops one week or more after entering an area where there is a malaria risk and up to 3 months (or, rarely, later) after departure from a risk area.

Protection against mosquito bites

All travellers should be advised that individual protection from mosquito bites between dusk and dawn is their first line of defence against malaria. Practical measures for protection are described in Chapter 3, in the section "Protection against vectors".

Chemoprophylaxis

The most appropriate chemoprophylactic antimalarial drug(s) (if any) for the destination(s) should be prescribed in the correct dosages (see Country list and Table 7.1).

Travellers and their doctors should be aware that

NO ANTIMALARIAL PROPHYLACTIC REGIMEN GIVES COMPLETE PROTECTION,

but good chemoprophylaxis (adherence to the recommended drug regimen) does reduce the risk of fatal disease. The following should also be taken into account:

- Dosing schedules for children should be based on body weight.
- Antimalarials that have to be taken daily should be started the day before arrival in the risk area.
- Weekly chloroquine should be started 1 week before arrival.

- Weekly mefloquine should preferably be started 2–3 weeks before departure, to achieve higher pre-travel blood levels and to allow side-effects to be detected before travel so that possible alternatives can be considered.

- All prophylactic drugs should be taken with unfailing regularity for the duration of the stay in the malaria risk area, and should be continued for 4 weeks after the last possible exposure to infection, since parasites may still emerge from the liver during this period. The single exception is atovaquone–proguanil, which can be stopped 1 week after return because of its effect on early liver-stage parasites ("liver schizonts").

- Depending on the predominant type of malaria at the destination, travellers should be advised about possible late-onset *P. vivax* and *P. ovale*.

Depending on the malaria risk in the area visited (see Country list), the recommended prevention method may be mosquito bite prevention only, or mosquito bite prevention in combination with chemoprophylaxis, as follows:

See Table 7.1 for details on individual drugs.

	Malaria risk	Type of prevention
Type I	Very limited risk of malaria transmission	Mosquito bite prevention only
Type II	Risk of *P. vivax* malaria only; or fully chloroquine-sensitive *P. falciparum*	Mosquito bite prevention plus chloroquine chemoprophylaxis
Type III	Risk of *P. vivax* and *P. falciparum* malaria transmission, combined with emerging chloroquine resistance	Mosquito bite prevention plus chloroquine+proguanil chemoprophylaxis
Type IV	(1) High risk of *P. falciparum* malaria, in combination with reported antimalarial drug resistance; or (2) Moderate/low risk of *P. falciparum* malaria, in combination with reported high levels of drug resistance	Mosquito bite prevention plus mefloquine, doxycycline or atovaquone–proguanil chemoprophylaxis (select according to reported resistance pattern)

All antimalarial drugs have specific contraindications and possible side-effects. Adverse reactions attributed to malaria chemoprophylaxis are common, but most are minor and do not affect the activities of the traveller. Serious adverse events – defined as constituting an apparent threat to life, requiring or prolonging hospitalization, or resulting in persistent or significant disability or incapacity – are rare and normally identified only when a drug has been in use for some time. Severe neuropsychiatric disturbances (seizures, psychosis, encephalopathy) occur in approximately 1 in 10 000 travellers receiving mefloquine prophylaxis. For malaria prophylaxis with atovaquone–proguanil or doxycycline, the risks of rare serious adverse events have not yet been established. The risk of drug-associated adverse events should be weighed against the risk of malaria, especially *P. falciparum* malaria, and local drug-resistance patterns.

Each of the antimalarial drugs is contraindicated in certain groups and individuals, and the contraindications should be carefully considered (see Table 7.1) to reduce the risk of serious adverse reactions. Pregnant women, people travelling with young children, and people with chronic illnesses should seek individual medical advice. Any traveller who develops serious side-effects to an antimalarial should stop taking the drug and seek immediate medical attention. This applies particularly to neurological or psychological disturbances experienced with mefloquine prophylaxis. Mild nausea, occasional vomiting or loose stools should not prompt discontinuation of prophylaxis, but medical advice should be sought if symptoms persist.

Long-term use of chemoprophylaxis

Adherence and tolerability are important aspects of chemoprophylaxis use in long-term travellers. There are few studies on chemoprophylaxis use in travel lasting more than 6 months. The risk of serious side-effects associated with long-term prophylactic use of chloroquine and proguanil is low, but retinal toxicity is of concern when a cumulative dose of 100 g of chloroquine is reached. Anyone who has taken 300 mg of chloroquine weekly for more than 5 years and requires further prophylaxis should be screened twice-yearly for early retinal changes. If daily doses of 100 mg chloroquine have been taken, screening should start after 3 years. Data indicate no increased risk of serious side-effects with long-term use of mefloquine if the drug is tolerated in the short-term. Available data on long-term chemoprophylaxis with doxycycline (i.e. more than 4–6 months) is limited but reassuring. Atovaquone–proguanil is registered in European countries with a restriction on duration of use (varying from 5 weeks to 3 months); in the USA no such restrictions apply.

Treatment

Early diagnosis and appropriate treatment can be life-saving. A blood sample should be taken from all (returning) travellers with suspected malaria and examined for malaria parasites. If no parasites are found in the first blood film, a series of blood samples should be taken at 6–12-hour intervals and examined very carefully. Malaria rapid diagnostic tests may be useful in centres where malaria microscopy is unavailable. When laboratory analysis is delayed, physicians should begin treatment if the clinical indicators and travel history suggest malaria.

For returning travellers who are treated for malaria in non-endemic areas, the following principles apply:

- Patients are at high risk of malaria and its consequences because they are non-immune.

- Effective medicines should be used.

- The prevention of emergence of resistance is of less relevance outside malaria-endemic areas. Thus monotherapy (e.g. with artesunate) may be given as long as the complete course of 7 days is taken.

- If the patient has taken prophylaxis, the same medicine should not be used for treatment.

The following antimalarials are suitable for treatment of **uncomplicated falciparum malaria** in travellers returning to non-endemic countries:

- artemether–lumefantrine
- atovaquone–proguanil
- quinine plus doxycycline or clindamycin.

The treatment for **vivax malaria** in travellers is as follows:

- Chloroquine plus primaquine is the treatment of choice.

- Amodiaquine combined with primaquine should be given for chloroquine-resistant vivax malaria.

- Travellers must be tested for glucose-6-phosphate dehydrogenase (G6PD) deficiency before receiving primaquine. In moderate G6PD deficiency, primaquine should be given in an adjusted regimen of 0.75 mg base/kg body weight once a week for 8 weeks. In severe G6PD deficiency, primaquine should not be given.

- In mixed *P. falciparum–P. vivax* infections, the treatment for *P. falciparum* will usually also cure the attack of *P. vivax*, but primaquine should be added to achieve radical cure and prevent relapses.

Relapsing malaria caused by *P. ovale* should be treated with chloroquine and primaquine. **Malaria caused by *P. malariae*** should be treated with the standard regimen of chloroquine as for vivax malaria, but it does not require radical cure with primaquine because no hypnozoites are formed in infection with this species.

Returning travellers with **severe falciparum malaria** should be managed in an intensive care unit. Parenteral antimalarial treatment should be with artesunate (first choice), artemether or quinine. If only parenteral quinidine is available, this should be given with careful clinical and electrocardiographic monitoring.

The dosage regimens for the treatment of uncomplicated malaria are provided in Table 7.2. The details of the clinical management of severe malaria are addressed in other WHO publications (see list of references).

Treatment abroad and stand-by emergency treatment

An individual who experiences a fever 1 week or more after entering an area of malaria risk should consult a physician or qualified malaria laboratory immediately to obtain a correct diagnosis and safe and effective treatment. In principle, travellers can be treated with artemisinin-based combination therapy (ACT) according to the national policy in the country they will be visiting. National antimalarial drug policies for all endemic countries are listed at http://www.who.int/malaria/treatmentpolicies.html

In light of the spread of counterfeit drugs in some resource-poor settings, travellers may opt to buy a reserve antimalarial treatment before departure, so that they can be confident of drug quality should they become ill.

Many travellers will be able to obtain proper medical attention within 24 hours of the onset of fever. For others, however, this may be impossible, particularly if they will be staying in remote locations. In such cases, travellers are advised to carry antimalarial drugs for self-administration ("stand-by emergency treatment").

Stand-by emergency treatment (SBET) may also be indicated for travellers in some occupational groups, such as aircraft crews, who make frequent short stops in endemic areas over a prolonged period of time. Such travellers may choose to reserve chemoprophylaxis for high-risk areas and seasons only. However, they should continue to take measures to protect against mosquito bites and be prepared for an attack of malaria: they should always carry a course of antimalarial drugs for SBET, seek immediate medical care in case of fever, and take SBET if prompt medical help is not available.

Furthermore, SBET – combined with protection against mosquito bites – may be indicated for those who travel for 1 week or more to remote rural areas where there is multidrug-resistant malaria but a very low risk of infection, and the risk of side-effects of prophylaxis may outweigh that of contracting malaria. This may be the case in certain border areas of Thailand and neighbouring countries in south-east Asia, as well as parts of the Amazon basin.

Studies on the use of rapid diagnostic tests ("dipsticks") have shown that untrained travellers experience major problems in the performance and interpretation of these tests, with an unacceptably high number of false-negative results. In addition, dipsticks can be degraded by extremes of heat and humidity, becoming less sensitive.

Successful SBET depends crucially on travellers' behaviour, and health advisers need to spend time explaining the strategy. Travellers provided with SBET should be given clear and precise written instructions on the recognition of symptoms, when and how to take the treatment, possible side-effects, and the possibility of drug failure. If several people travel together, the individual dosages for SBET should be specified. **Travellers should realize that self-treatment is a first-aid measure, and that they should still seek medical advice as soon as possible.**

In general, travellers carrying SBET should observe the following guidelines:

- Consult a physician immediately if fever occurs 1 week or more after entering an area with malaria risk.

- If it is impossible to consult a physician and/or establish a diagnosis within 24 hours of the onset of fever, start the stand-by emergency treatment and seek medical care as soon as possible for complete evaluation and to exclude other serious causes of fever.

- Do not treat suspected malaria with the same drugs used for prophylaxis.

- Vomiting of antimalarial drugs is less likely if fever is first lowered with antipyretics. A second full dose should be taken if vomiting occurs within 30 minutes of taking the drug. If vomiting occurs 30–60 minutes after a dose, an additional half-dose should be taken. Vomiting with diarrhoea may lead to treatment failure because of poor drug absorption.

- Complete the stand-by treatment course and resume antimalarial prophylaxis 1 week after the *first* treatment dose. To reduce the risk of drug interactions, at least 12 hours should elapse between the *last* treatment dose of quinine and resumption of mefloquine prophylaxis.

The drug options for SBET are in principle the same as for treatment of uncomplicated malaria (see above). The choice will depend on the type of malaria in the area visited and the chemoprophylaxis regimen taken. Artemether–lumefantrine has been registered (in Switzerland and the United Kingdom) for use as SBET for travellers. Table 7.2 provides details on individual drugs.

Multidrug-resistant malaria

Multidrug-resistant malaria has been reported from south-east Asia (Cambodia, Myanmar, Thailand, Viet Nam) and the Amazon basin of South America, where it occurs in parts of Brazil, French Guiana and Suriname.

In border areas between Cambodia, Myanmar and Thailand, *P. falciparum* infections do not respond to treatment with chloroquine or sulfadoxine–pyrimethamine, sensitivity to quinine is reduced, and treatment failures in excess of 50% with mefloquine are being reported. In these situations, malaria prevention consists of personal protection measures in combination with atovaquone–proguanil or doxycycline as chemoprophylaxis. SBET with atovaquone–proguanil or artemether–lumefantrine can be used in situations where the risk of infection is very low. However, these drugs cannot be given to pregnant women and young children. Since there is no prophylactic or SBET regimen that is both effective and safe for these groups in areas of multidrug-resistant malaria, pregnant women and young children should avoid travelling to these malarious areas.

Special groups

Some groups of travellers, especially young children and pregnant women, are at particular risk of serious consequences if they become infected with malaria. Recommendations for these groups are difficult to formulate because safety data are limited.

Pregnant women

Malaria in a pregnant woman increases the risk of maternal death, miscarriage, stillbirth and low birth weight with associated risk of neonatal death.

Pregnant women should be advised to avoid travelling to areas where malaria transmission occurs. When travel cannot be avoided, it is very important to take effective preventive measures against malaria, even when travelling to areas with transmission only of vivax malaria. Pregnant women should seek medical help immediately if malaria is suspected; if this is not possible, they should take stand-by emergency treatment. Medical help must be sought as soon as possible after starting stand-by treatment. There is very limited information on the safety and efficacy of most antimalarials in pregnancy, particularly during the first trimester. However, inadvertent exposure to antimalarials is not an indication for termination of the pregnancy.

Mosquito bite prevention
Pregnant women should be extra diligent in using measures to protect against mosquito bites, including insect repellents and insecticide-treated mosquito nets. They should take care not to exceed the recommended dosage of insect repellents.

Chemoprophylaxis
In type II areas, with exclusively *P. vivax* transmission or where *P. falciparum* can be expected to be fully sensitive to chloroquine, prophylaxis with chloroquine alone may be used. In type III areas, prophylaxis with chloroquine plus proguanil can be safely prescribed, including during the first 3 months of pregnancy. In type IV areas, mefloquine prophylaxis may be given during the second and third trimesters, but there is limited information on the safety of mefloquine during the first trimester. In light of the danger of malaria to mother and fetus, experts increasingly agree that travel to a chloroquine-resistant *P. falciparum* area during the first trimester of pregnancy should be avoided or delayed at all costs; if this is truly impossible, good preventive measures should be taken, including prophylaxis with mefloquine where this is indicated. Doxycycline is contraindicated during pregnancy. Atovaquone–proguanil has not been sufficiently investigated to be prescribed in pregnancy.

Treatment
Clindamycin and quinine are considered safe, including during the first trimester of pregnancy; artemisinin derivatives can be used to treat uncomplicated malaria in the second and third trimesters, and in the first trimester only if no other adequate medicines are available. Amodiaquine and chloroquine can be safely used for treatment of vivax malaria in pregnancy, but primaquine anti-relapse treatment should be postponed until after delivery. Atovaquone–proguanil and artemether–lumefantrine have not been sufficiently investigated to be prescribed in pregnancy.

The recommended treatment for uncomplicated falciparum malaria in the first trimester is quinine +/– clindamycin. For the second and third trimesters, the options are: ACT in accordance with national policy; artesunate +/– clindamycin; or quinine +/– clindamycin.

Pregnant women with falciparum malaria, particularly in the second and third trimesters of pregnancy, are more likely than other adults to develop severe malaria, often complicated by hypoglycaemia and pulmonary oedema. Maternal mortality in severe malaria is approximately 50%, which is higher than in non-pregnant adults. Fetal death and premature labour are common. Pregnant women with severe malaria must be treated without delay with full doses of parenteral antimalarial treatment. Where available, artesunate is the first option and arte-mether the second for the management of severe malaria in the second and third trimesters. Until more evidence becomes available, both artesunate and quinine may be considered as options in the first trimester. Treatment must not be delayed, so if only one of the drugs artesunate, artemether, or quinine is available it should be started immediately.

Information on the safety of antimalarial drugs during breastfeeding is provided in Tables 7.1 and 7.2.

Women who may become pregnant during or after travel

Both mefloquine and doxycycline prophylaxis may be taken but pregnancy should preferably be avoided during the period of drug intake and for 3 months after mefloquine and 1 week after doxycycline prophylaxis is stopped. If pregnancy occurs during antimalarial prophylaxis with mefloquine or doxycycline, this is not considered to be an indication for pregnancy termination. Because its half-life in adults is 2–3 days, more than 99% of atovaquone will usually be eliminated from the body by 3 weeks after the last dose was taken.

Young children

Falciparum malaria in a young child is a medical emergency. It may be rapidly fatal. Early symptoms are atypical and difficult to recognize, and life-threatening complications can occur within hours of the initial symptoms. Medical help should be sought immediately if a child develops a febrile illness within 3 months (or, rarely, later) of travelling to an endemic area. Laboratory confirmation of diagnosis should be requested immediately, and treatment with an effective antimalarial drug initiated as soon as possible. In infants, malaria should be suspected even in non-febrile illness.

Parents should be advised not to take babies or young children to areas with risk of falciparum malaria. If travel cannot be avoided, children must be very carefully protected against mosquito bites and be given appropriate chemoprophylactic drugs.

Mosquito bite prevention

Babies should be kept under insecticide-treated mosquito nets as much as possible between dusk and dawn. The manufacturer's instructions on the use of insect repellents should be followed diligently, and the recommended dosage must not be exceeded.

Chemoprophylaxis

Breastfed, as well as bottle-fed, babies should be given chemoprophylaxis since they are not protected by the mother's prophylaxis. Dosage schedules for children should be based on body weight, and tablets should be crushed and ground as necessary. The bitter taste of the tablets can be disguised with jam or other foods. Chloroquine and proguanil are safe for babies and young children but their use is now very limited, because of spreading chloroquine resistance. Mefloquine may be given to infants of more than 5 kg body weight. Atovaquone–proguanil is generally not recommended for prophylaxis in children who weigh less than 11 kg, because of limited data; in the USA it is given for prophylaxis in infants of more than 5 kg body weight. Doxycycline is contraindicated in children below 8 years of age. All antimalarial drugs should be kept out of the reach of children and stored in childproof containers: chloroquine is particularly toxic in case of overdose.

Treatment

Acutely ill children with falciparum malaria require careful clinical monitoring as they may deteriorate rapidly. Every effort should be made to give oral treatment and ensure that it is retained. ACT as per national policy can be used as first-line treatment while abroad. Oral treatment options for SBET and returning travellers are: artemether-lumefantrine (not recommended under 5 kg because of lack of data), atovaquone–proguanil (apparently safe in children weighing 5 kg or more, but limited data), and quinine plus clindamycin (safe, but limited data on clindamycin). Quinine plus doxycycline is an option for children of 8 years and older. Parenteral treatment and admission to hospital are indicated for young children who cannot swallow antimalarials reliably.

Chloroquine and amodiaquine can be safely given to treat *P. vivax, P. ovale* or *P. malariae* infections in young children. The lower age limit for anti-relapse treatment with primaquine has not been established; it is generally contraindicated in young infants.

Information on the safety of drugs for prophylaxis and treatment of young children is provided in Tables 7.1 and 7.2.

HIV/AIDS

Immunosuppressed travellers are at increased risk of malaria, and prevention of malaria through avoidance of mosquito bites and use of chemoprophylaxis is particularly important. Individual pre-travel advice should be sought, and should also avoid possible drug interactions between antiretroviral and antimalarial drugs. There may be an increased risk of antimalarial treatment failure in people living with HIV/AIDS at present, however, there is insufficient information to permit modifications to treatment regimens to be recommended. Cutaneous drug reactions following treatment with sulfadoxine–pyrimethamine are more common in people infected with HIV. Treatment with ACT containing sulfadoxine–pyrimethamine should be avoided in HIV-infected patients receiving co-trimoxazole prophylaxis.

Table 7.1 **Use of antimalarial drugs for prophylaxis in travellers**

| Generic name | Dosage regimen | Duration of prophylaxis | Use in special groups | | | Main contraindications[a] | Comments[a] |
			Pregnancy	Breast-feeding	Children		
Atovaquone–proguanil combination tablet	One dose daily. *11–20 kg*: 62.5 mg atovaquone plus 25 mg proguanil (1 paediatric tablet) daily *21–30 kg*: 2 paediatric tablets daily *31–40 kg*: 3 paediatric tablets daily *>40 kg*: 1 adult tablet (250 mg atovaquone plus 100 mg proguanil) daily	Start 1 day before departure and continue for 7 days after return	No data, not recommended	No data, not recommended	Not recommended under 11 kg because of limited data	Hypersensitivity to atova-quone and/or proguanil; severe renal insufficiency (creatinine clearance <30 ml/min).	Registered in European countries for chemoprophylactic use with a restriction on duration of use (varying from 5 weeks to 3 months). Plasma concentrations of atovaquone are reduced when it is co-administered with rifampicin, rifabutin, metoclopramide or tetracycline.
Chloroquine	5 mg base/kg weekly in one dose, or 10 mg base/kg weekly divided in 6 daily doses *Adult dose*: 300 mg chloroquine base weekly in one dose, or 600 mg chloroquine base weekly divided over 6 daily doses of 100 mg base (with one drug-free day per week)	Start 1 week before departure and continue for 4 weeks after return. If daily doses: start 1 day before departure	Safe	Safe	Safe	Hypersensitivity to chloroquine; history of epilepsy; psoriasis.	Concurrent use of chloroquine can reduce the antibody response to intradermally administered human diploid-cell rabies vaccine.
Chloroquine–proguanil combination tablet	*>50 kg*: 100 mg chloroquine base plus 200 mg proguanil (1 tablet) daily	Start 1 day before departure and continue for 4 weeks after return	Safe	Safe	Tablet size not suitable for persons of < 50 kg body weight	Hypersensitivity to chloroquine and/or proguanil; liver or kidney insufficiency; history of epilepsy; psoriasis.	Concurrent use of chloroquine can reduce the antibody response to intradermally administered human diploid-cell rabies vaccine.

[a] Please see package insert for full information on contraindications and precautions.

Table 7.1 Use of antimalarial drugs for prophylaxis in travellers (*continued*)

Generic name	Dosage regimen	Duration of prophylaxis	Use in special groups			Main contraindications[a]	Comments[a]
			Pregnancy	Breast-feeding	Children		
Doxycycline	1.5 mg salt/kg daily *Adult dose*: 1 tablet of 100 mg daily	Start 1 day before departure and continue for 4 weeks after return	Contra-indicated	Contra-indicated	Contra-indicated under 8 years of age	Hypersensitivity to tetra-cyclines; liver dysfunction.	Doxycycline makes the skin more susceptible to sunburn. People with sensitive skin should use a highly protective (UVA) sunscreen and avoid prolonged direct sunlight, or switch to another drug. Doxycycline should be taken with plenty of water to prevent oesophageal irritation. Doxycycline may increase the risk of vaginal *Candida* infections. Studies indicate that the monohydrate form of the drug is better tolerated than the hyclate.
Mefloquine	5 mg/kg weekly *Adult dose*: 1 tablet of 250 mg weekly	Start at least 1 week (preferably 2–3 weeks) before departure and continue for 4 weeks after return	Not recom-mended in first tri-mester because of lack of data	Safe	Not recom-mended under 5 kg because of lack of data	Hypersensitivity to mefloquine; psychiatric (including depres-sion) or convulsive disorders; history of severe neuropsychia-tric disease; concomitant halofantrine treatment; treat-ment with mefloquine in previous 4 weeks; not recom-mended in view of limited data for people performing activities requiring fine coordination and spatial discrimination, e.g. pilots, machine operators.	Do not give mefloquine within 12 hours of quinine treatment. Mefloquine and other cardioactive drugs may be given concomitantly only under close medical supervision. Ampicillin, tetracycline and metoclopramide can increase mefloquine blood levels.
Proguanil	3 mg/kg daily *Adult dose*: 2 tablets of 100 mg daily	Start 1 day before departure and continue for 4 weeks after return	Safe	Safe	Safe	Liver or kidney dysfunction.	Use only in combination with chloroquine. Proguanil can interfere with live typhoid vaccine.

[a] Please see package insert for full information on contraindications and precautions.

161

Table 7.2 **Use of antimalarial drugs for treatment of uncomplicated malaria in travellers**

Generic name	Dosage regimen	Duration of prophylaxis	Use in special groups[a]			Main contraindications[a]	Comments[a]
			Pregnancy	Breast-feeding	Children		
Amodiaquine	30 mg base/kg taken as 10 mg base/kg for 3 days		Apparently safe but limited data	Apparently safe but limited data	Safe	Hypersensitivity to amodiaquine; hepatic disorders.	Use only for malaria caused by *P. vivax*, *P. ovale* or *P. malariae*.
Artemether-lumefantrine combination tablet	3-day course of 6 doses total, taken at 0, 8, 24, 36, 48, and 60 hours 5–14 kg: 1 tablet (20 mg artemether plus 120 mg lumefantrine) per dose 15–24 kg: 2 tablets per dose 25–34 kg: 3 tablets per dose 35 kg and over: 4 tablets per dose		No data, not recommen-ded	No data, not recommen-ded	Not recom-mended under 5 kg because of lack of data	Hypersensitivity to artemether and/or lumefantrine.	Better absorbed if taken with fatty foods.
Artemisinin and derivatives	*Artemisinin:* 10 mg/kg daily for 7 days *Artemisinin derivatives:* 2 mg/kg daily for 7 days Artemisinin and its derivatives are given with a double divided dose on the first day		Not recom-mended in first trimester because of lack of data	Safe	Safe	Hypersensitivity to artemisinins.	Normally taken in combination with another effective antimalarial (as ACT), which reduces the duration of treatment to 3 days. As monotherapy, these drugs should be taken for a minimum of 7 days, to prevent recrudescences.
Atovaquone-proguanil combination tablet	One dose daily for 3 consecutive days 5–8 kg: 2 paediatric tablets daily (at 62.5 mg atovaquone plus 25 mg proguanil per tablet) 9–10 kg: 3 paediatric tablets daily 11–20 kg: 1 adult tablet (250 mg atovaquone plus 100 mg proguanil) daily 21–30 kg: 2 adult tablets daily 31–40 kg: 3 adult tablets daily > 40 kg: 4 adult tablets (1 g atovaquone plus 400 mg proguanil) daily		No data, not recommen-ded	No data, not recommen-ded	Apparently safe in children > 5 kg, but limited data	Hypersensitivity to atovaquone and/or proguanil; severe renal insufficiency (creatinine clearance <30 ml/min).	Plasma concentrations of atovaquone are reduced when the drug is co-administered with rifampicin, rifabutin, metoclopramide or tetracycline.

[a] Please see package insert for full information on contraindications and precautions.

Table 7.2 Use of antimalarial drugs for treatment of uncomplicated malaria in travellers (*continued*)

Generic name		Use in special groups			Main contraindications[a]	Comments[a]
	Dosage regimen	Duration of prophylaxis	Pregnancy	Breast-feeding	Children		

Generic name	Dosage regimen	Duration of prophylaxis	Pregnancy	Breast-feeding	Children	Main contraindications[a]	Comments[a]
Chloroquine	25 mg base/kg divided in daily dose (10, 10, 5 mg base/kg) for 3 days	Safe	Safe	Safe	Safe	Hypersensitivity to chloroquine; history of epilepsy; psoriasis.	Use only for malaria caused by *P. vivax*, *P. ovale* or *P. malariae*. Concurrent use of chloroquine can reduce the antibody response to intradermally administered human diploid-cell rabies vaccine.
Clindamycin	*Under 60 kg:* 5 mg base/kg 4 times daily for 5 days *60 kg and over:* 300 mg base 4 times daily for 5 days		Apparently safe but limited data	Apparently safe but limited data	Apparently safe but limited data	Hypersensitivity to clindamycin or lincomycin; history of gastrointestinal disease, particularly colitis; severe liver or kidney impairment.	Used in combination with quinine in areas of emerging quinine resistance.
Doxycycline	*Adults >50 kg:* 800 mg salt over 7 days, taken as 2 tablets (100 mg salt each) 12 hours apart on day 1, followed by 1 tablet daily for 6 days *Children 8 years and older:* 25–35 kg: 0.5 tablet per dose 36–50 kg: 0.75 tablet per dose > 50 kg: 1 tablet per dose	Contra-indicated	Contra-indicated	Contra-indicated	Contra-indicated under 8 years of age	Hypersensitivity to tetracyclines; liver dysfunction.	Used in combination with quinine in areas of emerging quinine resistance.

[a] Please see package insert for full information on contraindications and precautions.

163

Table 7.2 Use of antimalarial drugs for treatment of uncomplicated malaria in travellers (continued)

Generic name	Dosage regimen	Duration of prophylaxis	Use in special groups			Comments[a]
			Pregnancy	Breast-feeding	Children	
Mefloquine	25 mg base/kg as split dose (15 mg/kg plus 10 mg/kg 6–24 hours apart)	Not recommended in first trimester because of lack of data	Safe	Safe	Not recommended under 5 kg because of lack of data	Hypersensitivity to mefloquine; psychiatric (including depression) or convulsive disorders; history of severe neuropsychiatric disease; concomitant halofantrine treatment; treatment with mefloquine in previous 4 weeks; use with caution in people whose activities require fine coordination and spatial discrimination, e.g. pilots and machine operators.	Do not give mefloquine within 12 hours of last dose of quinine treatment. Mefloquine and other related compounds (such as quinine, quinidine, chloroquine) may be given concomitantly only under close medical supervision because of possible additive cardiac toxicity and increased risk of convulsions; co-administration of mefloquine with anti-arrhythmic agents, beta-adrenergic blocking agents, calcium channel blockers, antihistamines including H1-blocking agents, and phenothiazines may contribute to prolongation of QTc interval. Ampicillin, tetracycline and metoclopramide can increase mefloquine blood levels.
					Main contraindications[a]	
Primaquine	0.25 mg base/kg, taken with food once daily for 14 days In Oceania and South-East Asia the dose should be 0.5 mg base/kg	Contra-indicated	Safe		Lower age limit not established. Generally contraindicated in young infants	G6PD deficiency; active rheumatoid arthritis; lupus erythematosus; conditions that predispose to granulocytopenia; concomitant use of drugs that may induce haematological disorders.	Anti-relapse treatment of P. vivax and P. ovale infections.

[a] Please see package insert for full information on contraindications and precautions.

Table 7.2 Use of antimalarial drugs for treatment of uncomplicated malaria in travellers (continued)

Generic name	Dosage regimen	Duration of prophylaxis	Use in special groups		Main contraindications[a]	Comments[a]
			Pregnancy	Breast-feeding	Children		
Quinine	8 mg base/kg 3 times daily for 7 days	Safe	Safe	Safe	Hypersensitivity to quinine or quinidine; tinnitus; optic neuritis; haemolysis; myasthenia gravis. Use with caution in persons with G6PD deficiency and in patients with atrial fibrillation, cardiac conduction defects or heart block. Quinine may enhance effect of cardiosuppressant drugs. Use with caution in persons using beta-blockers, digoxin, calcium channel blockers, etc.	In areas of high-level resistance to quinine, give in combination with doxycycline, tetracycline or clindamycin. Quinine may induce hypoglycaemia, particularly in (malnourished) children, pregnant women and patients with severe disease.

[a] Please see package insert for full information on contraindications and precautions.

Countries and territories with malarious areas

The following list shows all countries where malaria occurs. In some of these countries, malaria is present only in certain areas or up to a particular altitude. In many countries, malaria has a seasonal pattern. These details as well as information on the predominant malaria species, status of resistance to antimalarial drugs and recommended type of prevention are provided in the Country list.

(* = *P. vivax* risk only)

Afghanistan
Algeria*
Angola
Argentina*
Armenia*
Azerbaijan*
Bangladesh
Belize
Benin
Bhutan
Bolivia
Botswana
Brazil
Burkina Faso
Burundi
Cambodia
Cameroon
Cape Verde
Central African
    Republic
Chad
China
Colombia
Comoros
Congo
Congo, Democratic
    Republic of the
    (former Zaire)
Costa Rica
Côte d'Ivoire
Djibouti
Dominican Republic
Ecuador
Egypt
El Salvador
Equatorial Guinea
Eritrea
Ethiopia

French Guiana
Gabon
Gambia
Georgia*
Ghana
Guatemala
Guinea
Guinea-Bissau
Guyana
Haiti
Honduras
India
Indonesia
Iran, Islamic Republic of
Iraq*
Kenya
Korea, Democratic
    People's Republic of*
Korea, Republic of*
Kyrgyzstan*
Lao People's Democratic
    Republic
Liberia
Madagascar
Malawi
Malaysia
Mali
Mauritania
Mauritius*
Mayotte
Mexico
Morocco*
Mozambique
Myanmar
Namibia
Nepal
Nicaragua
Niger

Nigeria
Oman
Pakistan
Panama
Papua New Guinea
Paraguay*
Peru
Philippines
Rwanda
Sao Tome and Principe
Saudi Arabia
Senegal
Sierra Leone
Solomon Islands
Somalia
South Africa
Sri Lanka
Sudan
Suriname
Swaziland
Syrian Arab
    Republic*
Tajikistan
Tanzania, United
    Republic of
Thailand
Timor-Leste
Togo
Turkey*
Turkmenistan*
Uganda
Uzbekistan*
Vanuatu
Venezuela
Viet Nam
Yemen
Zambia
Zimbabwe

Further reading

Guidelines for the treatment of malaria. Geneva, World Health Organization, 2006 (WHO/HTM/MAL/2006.1108).

Malaria vector control and personal protection: report of a WHO Study Group. Geneva, World Health Organization, 2006 (WHO Technical Report Series, No. 936).

Management of severe malaria: a practical handbook, 2nd ed. Geneva, World Health Organization, 2000.

These documents are available on the WHO Global Malaria Programme web site: http://www.who.int/malaria.

CHAPTER 8

Exposure to blood or other body fluids

Blood transfusion

Blood transfusion is a life-saving intervention. When used correctly, it saves lives and improves health. However, blood transfusion carries a potential risk of acute or delayed complications and transfusion-transmitted infections and should be prescribed only to treat conditions associated with significant morbidity that cannot be prevented or managed effectively by other means.

For travellers, the need for a blood transfusion almost always arises as a result of a medical emergency involving sudden massive blood loss, such as:

- traffic accident
- gynaecological or obstetric emergency
- severe gastrointestinal haemorrhage
- emergency surgery.

The safety of blood and blood products depends on two key factors:

- A supply of safe blood and blood products through the careful selection of voluntary unpaid blood donors from low-risk populations, testing all donated blood for transfusion-transmissible infections and correct storage and transportation before transfusion with adequate quality system.

- The appropriate prescription (only when there is no other remedy) and safe administration of the blood or blood product, correctly cross-matched for the recipient.

In many developing countries, safe blood and blood products may not be available in all health care facilities. In addition, evidence from every region of the world indicates considerable variations in patterns of clinical blood use between different hospitals, different clinical specialties and even between different clinicians within the same team. This suggests that blood and blood products are often transfused unnecessarily.

While blood transfusions correctly given save millions of lives every year, unsafe blood transfusions – as a result of the incompatibility of the blood or the transmission of infections such as hepatitis B, hepatitis C, human immunodeficiency virus (HIV) malaria, syphilis or Chagas disease – can lead to serious complications in the recipient.

The initial management of major haemorrhage is the prevention of further blood loss and restoration of the blood volume as rapidly as possible in order to maintain tissue perfusion and oxygenation. This requires infusing the patient with large volumes of replacement fluids until control of haemorrhage can be achieved. Some patients respond quickly and remain stable following the infusion of crystalloids or colloids and may not require blood transfusion.

In malaria-endemic areas, there is a high risk of acquiring malaria from transfusion. It may be necessary to give the transfused patient routine treatment for malaria.

Precautions

- Travellers should carry a medical card or other document showing their blood group and information about any current medical problems or treatment.
- Unnecessary travel should be avoided by those with pre-existing conditions that may give rise to a need for blood transfusion.
- Travellers should take all possible precautions to avoid involvement in traffic accidents (see Chapter 4).
- Travellers should obtain a contact address at the travel destination, in advance, for advice and assistance in case of medical emergency.
- Travellers with chronic medical conditions, such as thalassaemia or haemophilia, that necessitate regular transfusion of blood or plasma-derived products should obtain medical advice on the management of their condition before travelling. They should also identify appropriate medical facilities at their travel destination and carry a supply of the relevant products with them, if appropriate.

Accidental exposure to blood or other body fluids

Exposure to bloodborne pathogens may occur in case of:

- contact with blood or body fluids with a non-intact skin or with mucous membranes;
- through percutaneous injury with needles or sharp instruments contaminated with blood or body fluids.

These exposures may occur:

- when using contaminated syringes and needles for injecting drugs;
- as a result of accidents or acts of violence, including sexual assaults;
- in case of sexual exposure if there was no condom use, or if the condom was broken;
- as occupational exposure, within and outside health care settings, to health care and other workers (such as rescuers, police officers) in the course of the work or to patients;
- during natural or man-made disasters.

Accidental exposure may lead to infection by bloodborne pathogens, particularly hepatitis B, hepatitis C and HIV. The average risk of seroconversion after a single percutaneous exposure to infected blood for hepatitis C is approximately 2% and for hepatitis B it is 6–60%. The average risk of seroconversion to HIV after a single percutaneous exposure to HIV-infected blood is 0.1–0.3%. The risk of transmission through exposure to infected fluids or tissues is believed to be lower than that through exposure to infected blood.

Pre-exposure vaccination: Hepatitis B vaccination can be given to protect travellers from hepatitis B infection prior to exposure (see Chapter 6). There are no vaccines for hepatitis C or HIV.

Post-exposure prophylaxis: Post-exposure prophylaxis (PEP) is an emergency medical response given to prevent the transmission of bloodborne pathogens after potential exposure. It is available for HIV and hepatitis B.

Accidental exposure to potentially infected blood or other body fluids is a medical emergency. The following measures should be taken without delay.

1. Refer to a service provider and report the accident.

2. First-aid care.

3. PEP, if applicable.

First-aid care management of exposure to bloodborne pathogens:

After percutaneous exposure
- Allow the wound to bleed freely.

- Do not squeeze or rub the injury site.

- Wash site immediately using soap or a mild solution that will not irritate the skin.

- If running water is not available, clean site with a gel or hand-cleaning solution.
- Do not use any strong solutions, such as bleach or iodine, as these may irritate the wound and make the injury worse.

After a splash of blood or body fluids onto unbroken skin
- Wash the area immediately with running water.
- If running water is not available, clean the area with a gel or hand-cleaning solution.
- **Do not** use strong disinfectants (chlorhexidine gluconate is the best choice).

After exposure of the eye:
- Irrigate exposed eye immediately with water or normal saline.
- Sit in a chair, tilt the head back and ask a person to gently pour water or normal saline over the eye, gently pulling the eyelids up and down to make sure the eye is cleaned thoroughly.
- If wearing contact lenses, leave them in place while irrigating, as they form a barrier over the eye and will help protect it. Once the eye has been cleaned, remove the contact lenses and clean them in the normal manner. This will make them safe to wear again.
- **Do not** use soap or disinfectant on the eye.

After exposure of the mouth:
- Spit the fluid out immediately.
- Rinse the mouth thoroughly, using water or normal saline, and spit out again. Repeat this process several times.
- **Do not** use soap or disinfectant in the mouth.
- In all cases, a health care worker should be contacted immediately.

Post-exposure prophylaxis

HIV
For HIV, PEP refers to a set of comprehensive services to prevent HIV infection in the exposed individual. These services include risk assessment and counselling, HIV testing based on informed consent and – according to the risk assessment

– the provision of short-term antiretroviral (ARV) drugs, with follow up and support. Repatriation should be discussed and, if necessary, carried out as soon as possible.

PEP should be started as soon as possible after the incident and ideally within 2–4 hours. The decision to provide ARV drugs depends on a number of factors, including the HIV status of the source individual, the nature of the body fluid involved, the severity of exposure and the period between the exposure and the beginning of treatment. PEP should not be given to people who test or are known to be HIV-positive.

The recommended PEP regimen is, in most cases, a combination of two ARV drugs that should be taken continuously for 28 days. In some instances, when drug resistance may be suspected in the source person, a third drug may be added. Expert consultation is especially important when exposure to drug-resistant HIV may have occurred. More information is obtainable at: www.who.int/hiv/topics/prophylaxis/en/.

If HIV testing has been done, subsequent tests should be repeated 6 weeks and 3 and 6 months following exposure. People who test positive at these stages should be offered psychological support and appropriate treatment when needed.

After accidental exposure, the exposed individual should not have unprotected sexual intercourse, or give blood until the 6-months post-exposure tests confirm that he or she is not seropositive. Women should avoid becoming pregnant during this period.

Hepatitis B
For those who may be exposed to hepatitis B virus, infection can be prevented before exposure through vaccination and after exposure through PEP. Recommended post-exposure management algorithms for testing and administration of hepatitis B vaccine and/or hepatitis B immune globulin should be followed.

Hepatitis C
There is no vaccine against hepatitis C virus. People exposed to hepatitis C virus can be screened for hepatitis C virus RNA at baseline, 4–6 weeks and 4–6 months after exposure.

Further reading

The clinical use of blood in general medicine, obstetrics, paediatrics, surgery and anaesthesia, trauma and burns. Geneva, World Health Organization, 2001.

Post-exposure prophylaxis for HIV: www.who.int/hiv/topics/prophylaxis/en/

CHAPTER 9

Special groups of travellers

According to the World Tourism Organization, approximately 26% of the 800 million international journeys in the year 2005 were for visits to friends and relatives and for religious purposes/pilgrimages. This chapter looks at the health considerations of immigrants visiting friends and relatives and of pilgrims.

Travel to visit friends and relatives

This section was prepared in collaboration with the International Society of Travel Medicine

According to the United Nations, international migration rose from 120 million in 1990 to 190 million in 2005. In many countries immigrants now constitute more than 20% of the population. Immigrants increasingly travel to their place of origin to visit friends and relatives (VFR), and VFR travel is now a major component of the more than 800 million international journeys that take place annually. The term "VFRs" generally refers to immigrants from a developing country to an industrialized country who subsequently return to their home countries for the purpose of visiting friends and relatives.

Compared with tourists to the same destinations, VFRs are at increased risk of travel-related diseases. These include – but are not limited to – malaria, hepatitis A and B, typhoid fever, rabies, tuberculosis, and the diseases normally preventable by routine childhood vaccination. For example, the global surveillance data of GeoSentinel (an international network of travel medicine providers) on returned travel patients show that eight times more VFR travellers than tourists present with malaria as their diagnosed illness. It is estimated that VFRs account for more than half the total imported malaria cases in Europe and North America.

The greater risk for VFRs is related to a number of factors, including higher risk of exposure and insufficient protective measures. These individuals are less likely to seek pre-travel advice or to be adequately vaccinated, but more likely to stay in remote rural areas, have close contact with local populations, consume high-risk food and beverages, undertake last-minute travel and make trips of greater duration. Risk awareness and risk perception also differ between VFRs and most tourist travellers, resulting in a lower uptake by VFRs of pre-travel vaccinations or malaria prophylaxis. The cost of pre-travel consultation, often not covered by health insurance programmes, may be onerous for VFRs, particular those with large families, and access to travel medicine services may be hampered by cultural and linguistic limitations.

Improving the access of VFRs to pre-travel health counselling is of increasing public health importance. Primary health care providers need to become more aware of the increased risks faced by VFRs. Strategies are needed to increase the awareness among VFRs of travel-related health risks and to facilitate uptake of pre-travel health advice, vaccinations and, where indicated, malaria prophylaxis.

Pilgrimage

Data for quantifying the risk of medical problems related to religious pilgrimages are limited. In terms of health risk, the best documented pilgrimage is the Hajj – the annual Muslim pilgrimage to Mecca and Medina in Saudi Arabia. During the Hajj, more than 2 million Muslims from all over the world congregate to perform their religious rituals. The resulting overcrowding has been associated with stampedes, traffic accidents and fire injuries. Cardiovascular disease is the most common cause of death. Heatstroke and severe dehydration are frequent when the Hajj season falls during the summer months.

Overcrowding also contributes to the potential dissemination of airborne infectious diseases or infections associated with person-to-person transmission during the Hajj. In 1987, an extensive outbreak of meningococcal disease serogroup A among pilgrims prompted the Saudi Arabian health authorities to introduce mandatory vaccination with bivalent A and C vaccine for all pilgrims. Following outbreaks of meningococcal disease serogroup W-135 in 2000 and 2001, all pilgrims must now be given the quadrivalent meningococcal vaccine (protecting against serogroups A, C, Y and W-135) and Hajj visas cannot be issued without proof of vaccination. The most frequently reported complaints among pilgrims are upper respiratory symptoms. Influenza vaccination has been reported to reduce influenza-like illness among pilgrims and should be a highly recommended vaccination for all those making the Hajj. Pneumococcal vaccination should also be recommended for those over the age of 65 years and for those who would benefit from it because of underlying medical conditions (see Chapter 6).

Cholera has caused Hajj-related outbreaks in the past but not since 1989, following improvements to the water supply and sewage systems. Hepatitis A vaccination is recommended for non-immune pilgrims, and routine vaccinations (such as polio, tetanus, diphtheria, tetanus and hepatitis B – see Chapter 6) should be up to date. Yellow fever vaccine is a requirement for pilgrims coming from areas or countries with risk of transmission of yellow fever (see Annex 1).

Since 2005, the Ministry of Health of Saudi Arabia requires that all individuals under 15 years of age who travel to Saudi Arabia from polio-affected countries show proof of vaccination with oral polio vaccine (OPV) 6 weeks before application for entry visa (see also Chapter 6). Irrespective of previous immunization history, all such individuals arriving in Saudi Arabia will also receive oral polio vaccine at border points. In 2006, in addition to the above, all travellers from Afghanistan, India, Nigeria and Pakistan, regardless of age and previous immunization history, will also receive an additional dose of OPV upon arrival in Saudi Arabia.

Updates on requirements and recommendations for the annual Hajj pilgrimage can be found in the *Weekly Epidemiological Record* (available on line at www. who.int/wer/en).

Further reading

Ahmed QA, Arabi YM, Memish ZA. Health risks at the Hajj. *Lancet*, 2006, 367:1008–1015.

Information on GeoSentinel: www.istm.org/geosentinel/main.html

International migration and development. Report of the Secretary General. New York, United Nations, 2006 (A60/871)

Leder K et al. Illness in travelers visiting friends and relatives: a review of the GeoSentinel Surveillance Network. *Clinical Infectious Diseases*, 2006, 43(9):1185–1193.

Tourism highlights: 2006 edition. Madrid, World Tourism Organization, 2006; available at http://www.unwto.org/facts/menu.html

Trends in total migrant stock: the 2005 revision. Population Division, Department of Economic and Social Affairs, United Nations Secretariat. (Document available at: http://www.un.org/esa/population/publications/migration/UN_Migrant_Stock_Documentation_2005.pdf)

Country list[1]
Yellow fever vaccination requirements and recommendations; and malaria situation

Introduction

The information provided for each country includes the requirements for mandatory yellow fever vaccination, recommendations for yellow fever vaccination and details concerning the malaria situation and recommended prevention.

Yellow fever

The risk of yellow fever transmission depends on the presence of the virus in the country either in humans, in mosquitoes or in animals.

Under the terms of the revised International Health Regulations (2005) which enter into force in June 2007, the term «infected areas» will no longer apply with respect to yellow fever. WHO will determine those areas where «a risk of yellow fever transmission is present» based on the following criteria: yellow fever has been reported currently or in the past plus the presence of vectors and animal reservoirs.

Yellow fever vaccination

Yellow fever vaccination is carried out for two different purposes:

1) To prevent the international spread of the disease by *protecting countries* from the risk of importing or spreading the yellow fever virus. These are mandatory requirements established by the country.

   The countries that require proof of vaccination[2] are those where the disease may or may not occur and where the mosquito vector and potential non-human

---

[1] For the purpose of this publication, the term "country" covers countries, territories and areas.

[2] Please note that the requirements for vaccination of infants over 6 months of age by some countries are not in accordance with WHO's recommendations (see Chapter 6). Travellers should however be informed that the requirement exists for entry into the countries concerned.

primate hosts of yellow fever are present. Consequently, any importation of the virus by an infected traveller could result in its propagation and establishment, leading to a permanent risk of infection for the human population. Proof of vaccination is required for all travellers coming from countries with risk of yellow fever transmission including transit through such countries. The international yellow fever vaccination certificate becomes valid 10 days after vaccination and remains valid for a period of 10 years. Countries requiring yellow fever vaccination for entry do so in accordance with the International Health Regulations. Country requirements are subject to change at any time. The country list below provides information on yellow fever requirements as provided by the countries.

2) *To protect individual travellers* who may be exposed to yellow fever infection

As yellow fever is frequently fatal for those who have not been vaccinated, vaccination is recommended for all travellers (with few exceptions - see Chapter 6) visiting areas where there is a risk of yellow fever transmission.

The fact that a country has no mandatory requirement for vaccination does not imply that there is no risk of yellow fever transmission.

Annex 1 provides a summary list of countries with risk of yellow fever transmission as well as a list of countries that require yellow vaccination for entry.

Other diseases

Cholera. No country requires a certificate of vaccination against cholera as a condition for entry. For information on selective use of cholera vaccines, see Chapter 6.

Smallpox. Since the global eradication of smallpox was certified in 1980, WHO does not recommend smallpox vaccination for travellers.

Other infectious diseases. Information on the main infectious disease threats for travellers, their geographical distribution, and corresponding precautions are provided in Chapter 5. Chapter 6 provides information on vaccine-preventable diseases.

Malaria

General information about the disease, its geographical distribution and details of preventive measures are included in Chapter 7. Protective measures against mosquito bites are described in Chapter 3. Specific information for each country is provided in this section, including epidemiological details for all countries with malarious areas (geographical and seasonal distribution, altitude, predominant species, reported resistance). The recommended prevention is also indicated. The recommended prevention for each country is decided on the basis of the following factors: the risk of contracting malaria; the prevailing species of malaria parasites in the area; the level and spread of drug resistance reported from the country; and the possible risk of serious side-effects resulting from the use of the various prophylactic drugs. Where *Plasmodium falciparum* and *P. vivax* both occur, prevention of falciparum malaria takes priority.

The numbers I, II, III and IV refer to the type of prevention based on the table below.

	Malaria risk	Type of prevention
Type I	Very limited risk of malaria transmission	Mosquito bite prevention only
Type II	Risk of *P. vivax* malaria only; or fully chloroquine-sensitive *P. falciparum*	Mosquito bite prevention plus chloroquine chemoprophylaxis
Type III	Risk of *P. vivax* and *P. falciparum* malaria transmission, combined with emerging chloroquine resistance	Mosquito bite prevention plus chloroquine+proguanil chemoprophylaxis
Type IV	(1) High risk of *P. falciparum* malaria, in combination with reported antimalarial drug resistance; or (2) Moderate/low risk of *P. falciparum* malaria, in combination with reported high levels of drug resistance	Mosquito bite prevention plus mefloquine, doxycycline or atovaquone–proguanil chemoprophylaxis (select according to reported resistance pattern)

AFGHANISTAN

Yellow fever:

Country requirement: A yellow fever vaccination certificate is required from travellers coming from areas with risk of yellow fever transmission.

Yellow fever vaccine recommendation: no

Malaria: Malaria risk—*P. vivax* and *P. falciparum*—exists from May through November below 2000 m. *P. falciparum* resistant to chloroquine and sulfadoxine–pyrimethamine reported.

Recommended prevention: **IV**

ALBANIA

Yellow fever:

Country requirement: A yellow fever vaccination certificate is required from travellers over 1 year of age coming from areas with risk of yellow fever transmission.

Yellow fever vaccine recommendation: no

ALGERIA

Yellow fever:

Country requirement: A yellow fever vaccination certificate is required from travellers over 1 year of age coming from areas with risk of yellow fever transmission.

Yellow fever vaccine recommendation: no

Malaria: Malaria risk is limited. Small foci of local transmission (*P. vivax*) have been reported in the 6 southern and south-eastern wilayas (Adrar, El Oued, Ghardaia, Illizi, Ouargla, Tamanrasset). Isolated local *P. falciparum* transmission has been reported from the two southernmost wilayas in areas under influence of trans-Saharan migration. No indigenous cases reported in 2005.

Recommended prevention in risk areas: **I**

AMERICAN SAMOA

Yellow fever:

Country requirement: no

Yellow fever vaccine recommendation: no

ANDORRA

Yellow fever:

Country requirement: no

Yellow fever vaccine recommendation: no

ANGOLA

Yellow fever:

Country requirement: A yellow fever vaccination certificate is required from all travellers over 1 year of age.

Malaria: Malaria risk—predominantly due to *P. falciparum*—exists throughout the year in the whole country. Resistance to chloroquine and sulfadoxine–pyrimethamine reported.

Recommended prevention: **IV**

ANGUILLA

Yellow fever:

Country requirement: A yellow fever vaccination certificate is required from travellers over 1 year of age coming from areas with risk of yellow fever transmission.

Yellow fever vaccine recommendation: no

ANTIGUA AND BARBUDA

Yellow fever:

Country requirement: A yellow fever vaccination certificate is required from travellers over 1 year of age coming from areas with risk of yellow fever transmission.

Yellow fever vaccine recommendation: no

ARGENTINA

Yellow Fever:

Country requirement: No

Yellow fever vaccine recommendation: No. Vaccination is recommended for travellers visiting Iguaçu Falls

Malaria: Malaria risk—exclusively due to *P. vivax*—is very low and is confined to rural areas along the borders with Bolivia (lowlands of Jujuy and Salta provinces) and with Paraguay (lowlands of Corrientes and Misiones provinces).

Recommended prevention in risk areas: **II**

ARMENIA

Yellow fever:

Country requirement: no

Yellow fever vaccine recommendation: no

Malaria: Malaria risk—exclusively due to *P. vivax*—exists focally from June through October in some of the villages located in Ararat Valley, mainly in the Masis district. No risk in tourist areas. No indigenous cases reported in 2006.

Recommended prevention: **I**

AUSTRALIA

Yellow fever:

Country requirement: A yellow fever vaccination certificate is required from travellers over 1 year of age entering Australia within 6 days of having stayed overnight or longer in a country with risk of yellow fever transmission, as listed in the *Weekly Epidemiological Record*.

Yellow fever vaccine recommendation: no

AUSTRIA

Yellow fever:

Country requirement: no

Yellow fever vaccine recommendation: no

AZERBAIJAN

Yellow fever:

Country requirement: no

Yellow fever vaccine recommendation: no

Malaria: Malaria risk—exclusively due to *P. vivax*—exists from June through October in lowland areas, mainly in the area between the Kura and the Arax rivers.

Recommended prevention: **I**

AZORES *see* PORTUGAL

BAHAMAS

Yellow fever:

Country requirement: A yellow fever vaccination certificate is required from travellers over 1 year of age coming from areas with risk of yellow fever transmission.

Yellow fever vaccine recommendation: no

BAHRAIN

Yellow fever:

Country requirement: no

Yellow fever vaccine recommendation: no

BANGLADESH

Yellow fever:

Country requirement: Any person (including infants) who arrives by air or sea without a certificate is detained in isolation for a period of up to 6 days if arriving within 6 days of departure from an area with risk of yellow fever transmission or having been in transit in such an area, or having come by an aircraft that has been in an area with risk of yellow fever transmission and has not been disinsected in accordance with the procedure and formulation laid down in Schedule VI of the Bangladesh Aircraft (Public Health) Rules 1977 (First Amendment) or those recommended by WHO.

The following countries and areas are regarded as areas with risk of yellow fever transmission:

Africa: Angola, Benin, Burkina Faso, Burundi, Cameroon, Central African Republic, Chad, Congo, Côte d'Ivoire, Democratic Republic of the Congo, Equatorial Guinea, Ethiopia, Gabon, Gambia, Ghana, Guinea, Guinea-Bissau, Kenya, Liberia, Malawi, Mali, Mauritania, Niger, Nigeria, Rwanda, Sao Tome and Principe, Senegal, Sierra Leone, Somalia, Sudan (south of 15°N), Togo, Uganda, United Republic of Tanzania, Zambia.

America: Belize, Bolivia, Brazil, Colombia, Costa Rica, Ecuador, French Guiana, Guatemala, Guyana, Honduras, Nicaragua, Panama, Peru, Suriname, Trinidad and Tobago, Venezuela.

Note. When a case of yellow fever is reported from any country, that country is regarded by the Government of Bangladesh as an area with risk of yellow fever transmission and is added to the above list.

Yellow fever vaccine recommendation: no

Malaria: Malaria risk exists throughout the year in the whole country excluding Dhaka city. *P. falciparum* resistant to chloroquine and sulfadoxine–pyrimethamine reported.

Recommended prevention: **IV**

BARBADOS

Yellow fever:

Country requirement: A yellow fever vaccination certificate is required from travellers over 1 year of age coming from areas with risk of yellow fever transmission.

Yellow fever vaccine recommendation: no

BELARUS

Yellow fever:

Country requirement: no

Yellow fever vaccine recommendation: no

BELGIUM

Yellow fever:

Country requirement: no

Yellow fever vaccine recommendation: no

BELIZE

Yellow fever:

Country requirement: A yellow fever vaccination certificate is required from travellers coming from areas with risk of yellow fever transmission.

Yellow fever vaccine recommendation: no

Malaria: Malaria risk—almost exclusively due to *P. vivax*—exists in all districts but varies within regions. Risk is highest in Toledo and Stan Creek Districts; moderate in Corozal and Cayo; and low in Belize District and Orange Walk. No resistant *P. falciparum* strains reported.

Recommended prevention in risk areas: **II**

BENIN

Yellow fever:

Country requirement: A yellow fever vaccination certificate is required from all travellers over 1 year of age.

Malaria: Malaria risk—predominantly due to *P. falciparum*—exists throughout the year in the whole country. Resistance to chloroquine and sulfadoxine-pyrimethamine reported.

Recommended prevention: **IV**

BERMUDA

Yellow fever:

Country requirement: no

Yellow fever vaccine recommendation: no

BHUTAN

Yellow fever:

Country requirement: A yellow fever vaccination certificate is required from travellers coming from areas with risk of yellow fever transmission.

Yellow fever vaccine recommendation: no

Malaria: Malaria risk exists throughout the year in the southern belt of the country comprising five districts: Chhukha, Samchi, Samdrup Jonkhar, Geyleg-phug and Shemgang. *P. falciparum* re-

sistant to chloroquine and sulfadoxine–pyrimethamine reported.

Recommended prevention in risk areas: **IV**

BOLIVIA

Yellow fever:

Country requirement: A yellow fever vaccination certificate is required from travellers coming from areas with risk of yellow fever transmission.

Yellow fever vaccine recommendation: recommended for incoming travellers visiting risk areas such as the province of Beni, Cochabamba and Santa Cruz, and the subtropical part of La Paz province. This does not include the cities of La Paz or Sucre.

Malaria: Malaria risk—predominantly due to *P. vivax* (95%)—exists throughout the year in the whole country below 2500 m. Falciparum malaria occurs in Santa Cruz and in the northern departments of Beni and Pando, especially in the localities of Guayaramerín and Riberalta. *P. falciparum* resistant to chloroquine and sulfadoxine–pyrimethamine reported.

Recommended prevention in risk areas: **II;** in Beni, Pando and Santa Cruz, **IV.**

BOSNIA AND HERZEGOVINA

Yellow fever:

Country requirement: no

Yellow fever vaccine recommendation: no

BOTSWANA

Yellow fever:

Country requirement: A yellow fever vaccination certificate is required from travellers over 1 year of age coming from or having passed through areas with risk of yellow fever transmission.

Yellow fever vaccine recommendation: no

Malaria: Malaria risk—predominantly due to *P. falciparum*—exists from November to May/ June in the northern parts of the country: Boteti, Chobe, Ngamiland, Okavango, Tutume districts/ sub-districts. Chloroquine-resistant *P. falciparum* reported.

Recommended prevention in risk areas: **IV.**

BRAZIL

Yellow fever:
Country requirement: A yellow fever vaccination certificate is required from travellers over 9 months of age coming from areas with risk of yellow fever transmission, unless they are in possession of a waiver stating that immunization is contraindicated on medical grounds.

Yellow fever vaccine recommendation: Vaccination is recommended for travellers to areas in Brazil with risk of yellow fever transmission, including rural areas in the states of Acre, Amapá, Amazonas, Goiás, Maranhão, Mato Grosso, Mato Grosso do Sul, Pará, Rondônia, Roraima and Tocantins, and to areas in other states where transmission risk exists, including the entire state of Minas Gerais and specific areas of the states of Espirito Santo, Piaui, Bahia, São Paulo, Paraná, Santa Catarina and Rio Grande do Sul. The complete list of municipalities are available at www.saude.gov.br/svs. Vaccination is recommended for travellers visiting Iguaçu Falls. Coastal cities, including Rio de Janeiro, Sao Paulo, Salvador, Recife, and Fortaleza, are NOT areas with risk of yellow fever transmission.

Malaria: Malaria risk—*P. vivax* (78%), *P. falciparum* (22%)—is present in most forested areas below 900 m within the nine states of the "Legal Amazonia" region (Acre, Amapá, Amazonas, Maranhão (western part), Mato Grosso (northern part), Pará (except Belém City), Rondônia, Roraima and Tocantins). Transmission intensity varies from municipality to municipality, but is higher in jungle areas of mining, lumbering and agricultural settlements less than 5 years old, than in the urban areas, including in large cities such as Pôrto Velho, Boa Vista, Macapá, Manaus, Santarém, Rio Branco and Maraba, where the transmission occurs on the periphery of these cities. In the states outside "Legal Amazonia", malaria transmission risk is negligible or non-existent. Multidrug-resistant *P. falciparum* reported.

Recommended prevention in risk areas: **IV**.

BRITISH VIRGIN ISLANDS

Yellow fever:
Country requirement: no

Yellow fever vaccine recommendation: no

BRUNEI DARUSSALAM

Yellow fever:
Country requirement: A yellow fever vaccination certificate is required from travellers over 1 year of age coming from areas with risk of yellow fever transmission or having passed through areas partly or wholly at risk of yellow fever transmission within the preceding 6 days.

Yellow fever vaccine recommendation: no

BULGARIA

Yellow fever:
Country requirement: no

Yellow fever vaccine recommendation: no

BURKINA FASO

Yellow fever:
Country requirement: A yellow fever vaccination certificate is required from all travellers over 1 year of age.

Malaria: Malaria risk—predominantly due to *P. falciparum*—exists throughout the year in the whole country. Resistance to chloroquine and sulfadoxine—pyrimethamine reported.

Recommended prevention: **IV**

BURMA see MYANMAR

BURUNDI

Yellow fever:
Country requirement: A yellow fever vaccination certificate is required from all travellers over 1 year of age.

Yellow fever vaccine recommendation: yes

Malaria: Malaria risk—predominantly due to *P. falciparum*—exists throughout the year in the whole country. Resistance to chloroquine and sulfadoxine-pyrimethamine reported.

Recommended prevention: **IV**

CAMBODIA

Yellow fever:
Country requirement: A yellow fever vaccination certificate is required from travellers coming from areas with risk of yellow fever transmission.

Yellow fever vaccine recommendation: no

Malaria: Malaria risk—predominantly due to *P. falciparum*—exists throughout the year in the whole country except in Phnom Penh and close around Tonle Sap. Risk within the tourist area of Angkor Wat is limited. *P. falciparum* resistant to chloroquine and sulfadoxine–pyrimethamine reported. Resistance to mefloquine reported in western provinces near the Thai border.

Recommended prevention: **IV**

CAMEROON

Yellow fever:

Country requirement: A yellow fever vaccination certificate is required from all travellers over 1 year of age.

Malaria: Malaria risk—predominantly due to *P. falciparum*—exists throughout the year in the whole country. Resistance to chloroquine and sulfadoxine–pyrimethamine reported.

Recommended prevention: **IV**

CANADA

Yellow fever:

Country requirement: no

Yellow fever vaccine recommendation: no

CANARY ISLANDS *see* SPAIN

CAPE VERDE

Yellow fever:

Country requirement: A yellow fever vaccination certificate is required from travellers over 1 year of age coming from countries with risk of yellow fever transmission.

Yellow fever vaccine recommendation: no

Malaria: Limited malaria risk exists from September through November in São Tiago Island.

Recommended prevention: **I**

CAYMAN ISLANDS

Yellow fever:

Country requirement: no

Yellow fever vaccine recommendation: no

CENTRAL AFRICAN REPUBLIC

Yellow fever:

Country requirement: A yellow fever vaccination certificate is required from all travellers over 1 year of age.

Malaria: Malaria risk—predominantly due to *P. falciparum*—exists throughout the year in the whole country. Resistance to chloroquine and sulfadoxine–pyrimethamine reported.

Recommended prevention: **IV**

CHAD

Yellow fever:

Country requirement: A yellow fever vaccination certificate is required from travellers coming from areas with risk of yellow fever transmission.

Yellow fever vaccine recommendation: yes

Malaria: Malaria risk—predominantly due to *P. falciparum*—exists throughout the year in the whole country. Resistance to chloroquine and sulfadoxine-pyrimethamine reported.

Recommended prevention: **IV**

CHILE

Yellow fever:

Country requirement: no

Yellow fever vaccine recommendation: no

CHINA

Yellow fever:

Country requirement: A yellow fever vaccination certificate is required from travellers coming from areas with risk of yellow fever transmission.

Yellow fever vaccine recommendation: no

Malaria: Malaria risk—including *P. falciparum* malaria—occurs in Hainan and Yunnan. Chloroquine and sulfadoxine–pyrimethamine resistant *P. falciparum* reported. Limited risk of *P. vivax* malaria exists in southern and some central provinces, including Anhui, Henan, Hubei, and Jiangsu. The risk may be higher in areas of focal outbreaks. There is no malaria risk in urban areas nor in the densely populated plain areas, nor at altitudes above 1500 m.

Recommended prevention in risk areas: **II;** in Hainan and Yunnan, **IV**

CHINA, HONG KONG SAR

Yellow fever:

Country requirement: no

Yellow fever vaccine recommendation: no

CHINA, MACAO SAR

Yellow fever:

Country requirement: no

Yellow fever vaccine recommendation: no

CHRISTMAS ISLAND

(Indian Ocean)

Same requirements as mainland Australia.

Yellow fever vaccine recommendation: no

COLOMBIA

Yellow fever:

Country requirement: No

Yellow fever vaccination recommendation: recommended for travellers who visit the following areas considered to be at risk of yellow fever: middle valley of the Magdalena river, eastern and western foothills of the Cordillera Oriental from the frontier with Ecuador to that with Venezuela, Chocoano and Antioqueño, Urabá, foothills of the Sierra Nevada de Santa Narta, eastern plains (Orinoquia and Amazonia).

Malaria: Malaria risk—*P. falciparum* (38%), *P. vivax* (62%)—is high throughout the year in rural/jungle areas below 1 600 m, especially in municipalities of the regions of Amazonia, Orinoquía, Pacífico and Urabá-Bajo Cauca. Transmission intensity varies by department, with the highest risk in Antioquia, Chocó, Córdoba, Nariño and Valle del Cauca. Chloroquine-resistant *P. falciparum* exists in Amazonia, Pacífico and Urabá-Bajo Cauca. Resistance to sulfadoxine–pyrimethamine reported.

Recommended prevention in risk areas: **III**; Amazonia, Pacífico and Urabá-Bajo Cauca, **IV**.

COMOROS

Yellow fever:

Country requirement: No

Yellow fever vaccine recommendation: no

Malaria: Malaria risk—predominantly due to *P. falciparum*—exists throughout the year in the whole country. Resistance to chloroquine and sulfadoxine—pyrimethamine reported.

Recommended prevention: **IV**

CONGO

Yellow fever:

Country requirement: A yellow fever vaccination certificate is required from all travellers over 1 year of age.

Malaria: Malaria risk—predominantly due to *P. falciparum*—exists throughout the year in the whole country. Resistance to chloroquine and sulfadoxine–pyrimethamine reported.

Recommended prevention: **IV**

CONGO, DEMOCRATIC REPUBLIC OF THE

Yellow fever:

Country requirement: A yellow fever vaccination certificate is required from all travellers over 1 year of age.

Malaria: Malaria risk—predominantly due to *P. falciparum*—exists throughout the year in the whole country. Resistance to chloroquine and sulfadoxine–pyrimethamine reported.

Recommended prevention: **IV**

COOK ISLANDS

Yellow fever:

Country requirement: no

Yellow fever vaccine recommendation: no

COSTA RICA

Yellow fever:

Country requirement: no

Yellow fever vaccine recommendation: no

Malaria: Malaria risk—almost exclusively due to *P. vivax*—occurs throughout the year in the provinces of Limón and Puntarenas, with highest risk in the cantons/Guacimo, Limón, Matina and Talamanca (Limón Province) and Garabito (Puntarenas Province). Negligible or no risk of malaria transmission exists in the other cantons of the country.

Recommended prevention in risk areas: **II**

CÔTE D'IVOIRE

Yellow fever:

Country requirement: A yellow fever vaccination certificate is required from all travellers over 1 year of age.

Malaria: Malaria risk—predominantly due to *P. falciparum*—exists throughout the year in the whole country. Resistance to chloroquine and sulfadoxine–pyrimethamine reported.

Recommended prevention: **IV**

CROATIA
Yellow fever:
Country requirement: no

Yellow fever vaccine recommendation: no

CUBA
Yellow fever:
Country requirement: no

Yellow fever vaccine recommendation: no

CYPRUS
Yellow fever:
Country requirement: no

Yellow fever vaccine recommendation: no

CZECH REPUBLIC
Yellow fever:
Country requirement: no

Yellow fever vaccine recommendation: no

DEMOCRATIC PEOPLE'S REPUBLIC OF KOREA *see* KOREA, DEMOCRATIC PEOPLE'S REPUBLIC OF

DEMOCRATIC REPUBLIC OF THE CONGO *see* CONGO, DEMOCRATIC REPUBLIC OF THE

DENMARK
Yellow fever:
Country requirement: no

Yellow fever vaccine recommendation: no

DJIBOUTI
Yellow fever:
Country requirement: A yellow fever vaccination certificate is required from travellers over 1 year of age coming from areas with risk of yellow fever transmission.

Yellow fever vaccine recommendation: no

Malaria: Malaria risk—predominantly due to *P. falciparum*—exists throughout the year in the whole country. Resistance to chloroquine and sulfadoxine–pyrimethamine reported.

Recommended prevention: **IV**

DOMINICA
Yellow fever:
Country requirement: A yellow fever vaccination certificate is required from travellers over 1 year of age coming from areas with risk of yellow fever transmission.

Yellow fever vaccine recommendation: no

DOMINICAN REPUBLIC
Yellow fever:
Country requirement: no

Yellow fever vaccine recommendation: no

Malaria: Malaria risk—exclusively due to *P. falciparum*—exists throughout the year, especially in the western provinces and in La Altagracia province. Risk in other areas is low to negligible. There is no evidence of *P. falciparum* resistance to any antimalarial drug.

Recommended prevention in risk areas: **II**

ECUADOR
Yellow fever:
Country requirement: A yellow fever vaccination certificate is required from travellers over 1 year of age coming from areas with risk of yellow fever transmission. Nationals and residents of Ecuador are required to possess certificates of vaccination on their departure to an area with risk of yellow fever transmission.

Yellow fever vaccine recommendation: In the east of the Andes Mountains. No risk in the cities of Quito and Guayaquil, or the Galapagos Islands.

Malaria: Malaria risk—*P. falciparum* (23%), *P. vivax* (77%)—exists throughout the year below 1500 m, with moderate to high transmission risk in El Oro, Esmeraldas, Guayas, Los Rios, Manabi, Morona Santiago, Napo, Orellana, Pastaza, Pichincha and Sucumbios. There is no risk in Guayaquil or Quito. *P. falciparum* resistance to chloroquine and sulfadoxine–pyrimethamine reported.

Recommended prevention in risk areas: **IV**

EAST TIMOR *see* TIMOR LESTE

EGYPT
Yellow fever:
Country requirement: A yellow fever vaccination certificate is required from travellers over 1 year of age coming from areas with risk of yellow fever

transmission. The following countries and areas are regarded as areas with risk of yellow fever transmission; air passengers in transit coming from these countries or areas without a certificate will be detained in the precincts of the airport until they resume their journey:

Africa: Angola, Benin, Burkina Faso, Burundi, Cameroon, Central African Republic, Chad, Congo, Côte d'Ivoire, Democratic Republic of the Congo, Equatorial Guinea, Ethiopia, Gabon, Gambia, Ghana, Guinea, Guinea-Bissau, Kenya, Liberia, Mali, Niger, Nigeria, Rwanda, Sao Tome and Principe, Senegal, Sierra Leone, Somalia, Sudan (south of 15°N), Togo, Uganda, United Republic of Tanzania, Zambia.

America: Belize, Bolivia, Brazil, Colombia, Costa Rica, Ecuador, French Guiana, Guyana, Panama, Peru, Suriname, Trinidad and Tobago, Venezuela.

All arrivals from Sudan are required to possess either a vaccination certificate or a location certificate issued by a Sudanese official centre stating that they have not been in Sudan south of 15°N within the previous 6 days.

Yellow fever vaccine recommendation: no

Malaria: Very limited *P. falciparum* and *P. vivax* malaria risk may exist from June through October in El Faiyûm governorate (no indigenous cases reported since 1998).

Recommended prevention: **none**

EL SALVADOR

Yellow fever:

Country requirement: A yellow fever vaccination certificate is required from travellers over 6 months of age coming from areas with risk of yellow fever transmission.

Yellow fever vaccine recommendation: no

Malaria: Very low malaria risk—almost exclusively due to *P. vivax*—exists throughout the year in Santa Ana Province, in rural areas of migratory influence from Guatemala. Sporadic vivax malaria cases are reported from other parts of the country.

Recommended prevention in risk areas: **II**

EQUATORIAL GUINEA

Yellow fever:

Country requirement: A yellow fever vaccination certificate is required from travellers coming from areas with risk of yellow fever transmission.

Yellow fever vaccine recommendation: yes

Malaria: Malaria risk—predominantly due to *P. falciparum*—exists throughout the year in the whole country. Resistance to chloroquine and sulfadoxine–pyrimethamine reported.

Recommended prevention: **IV**

ERITREA

Yellow fever:

Country requirement: A yellow fever vaccination certificate is required from travellers coming from areas with risk of yellow fever transmission.

Yellow fever vaccine recommendation: no

Malaria: Malaria risk—predominantly due to *P. falciparum*—exists throughout the year in the whole country below 2200 m. There is no risk in Asmara. Resistance to chloroquine and sulfadoxine–pyrimethamine reported.

Recommended prevention: **IV**

ESTONIA

Yellow fever:

Country requirement: no

Yellow fever vaccine recommendation: no

ETHIOPIA

Yellow fever:

Country requirement: A yellow fever vaccination certificate is required from travellers over 1 year of age coming from areas with risk of yellow fever transmission.

Yellow fever vaccine recommendation: yes

Malaria: Malaria risk—predominantly due to *P. falciparum*—exists throughout the year in the whole country below 2000 m. *P. falciparum* resistance to chloroquine and sulfadoxine–pyrimethamine reported. There is no malaria risk in Addis Ababa.

Recommended prevention: **IV**

FALKLAND ISLANDS (MALVINAS)

Yellow fever:

Country requirement: no

Yellow fever vaccine recommendation: no

FAROE ISLANDS

Yellow fever:

Country requirement: no

Yellow fever vaccine recommendation: no

FIJI

Yellow fever:

Country requirement: A yellow fever vaccination certificate is required from travellers over 1 year of age entering Fiji within 10 days of having stayed overnight or longer in areas with risk of yellow fever transmission.

Yellow fever vaccine recommendation: no

FINLAND

Yellow fever:

Country requirement: no

Yellow fever vaccine recommendation: no

(THE) FORMER YUGOSLAV REPUBLIC OF MACEDONIA see MACEDONIA, THE FORMER YUGOSLAV REPUBLIC OF

FRANCE

Yellow fever:

Country requirement: no

Yellow fever vaccine recommendation: no

FRENCH GUIANA

Yellow fever:

Country requirement: A yellow fever vaccination certificate is required from all travellers over 1 year of age.

Malaria: Malaria risk—*P. falciparum* (80%), *P. vivax* (20%)—is high throughout the year in nine munici-palities of the territory bordering Brazil (Oiapoque river valley) and Suriname (Maroni river valley). In the other 13 municipalities transmission risk is low or negligible. Multidrug-resistant *P. falciparum* reported in areas influenced by Brazilian migration.

Recommended prevention in risk areas: **IV**

FRENCH POLYNESIA

Yellow fever:

Country requirement: A yellow fever vaccination certificate is required from travellers over 1 year of age coming from areas with risk of yellow fever transmission.

Yellow fever vaccine recommendation: no

GABON

Yellow fever:

Country requirement: A yellow fever vaccination certificate is required from all travellers over 1 year of age.

Malaria: Malaria risk—predominantly due to *P. falciparum*—exists throughout the year in the whole country. Resistance to chloroquine and sulfadoxine–pyrimethamine reported.

Recommended prevention: **IV**

GALAPAGOS ISLANDS see EQUADOR

GAMBIA

Yellow fever:

Vaccine requirement: A yellow fever vaccination certificate is required from travellers over 1 year of age arriving from areas with risk of yellow fever transmission.

Yellow fever vaccine recommendation: yes

Malaria: Malaria risk—predominantly due to *P. falciparum*—exists throughout the year in the whole country. Resistance to chloroquine and sulfadoxine–pyrimethamine reported.

Recommended prevention: **IV**

GEORGIA

Yellow fever:

Country requirement: no

Yellow fever vaccine recommendation: no

Malaria: Malaria risk—exclusively due to *P. vivax*—exists focally from July to October in the south-eastern part of the country.

Recommended prevention: **I**

GERMANY

Yellow fever:

Country requirement: no

Yellow fever vaccine recommendation: no

GHANA

Yellow fever:

Country requirement: A yellow fever vaccination certificate is required from all travellers.

Malaria: Malaria risk—predominantly due to *P. falciparum*—exists throughout the year in the whole country. Resistance to chloroquine and sulfadoxine–pyrimethamine reported.

Recommended prevention: **IV**

GIBRALTAR

Yellow fever:

Country requirement: no

Yellow fever vaccine recommendation: no

GREECE

Yellow fever:

Country requirement: no

Yellow fever vaccine recommendation: no

GREENLAND

Yellow fever:

Country requirement: no

Yellow fever vaccine recommendation: no

GRENADA

Yellow fever:

Country requirement: A yellow fever vaccination certificate is required from travellers over 1 year of age coming from areas with risk of yellow fever transmission.

Yellow fever vaccine recommendation: no

GUADELOUPE

Yellow fever:

Country requirement: A yellow fever vaccination certificate is required from travellers over 1 year of age coming from areas with risk of yellow fever transmission.

Yellow fever vaccine recommendation: no

GUAM

Yellow fever:

Country requirement: no

Yellow fever vaccine recommendation: no

GUATEMALA

Yellow fever:

Country requirement: A yellow fever vaccination certificate is required from travellers over 1 year of age coming from countries with areas with risk of yellow fever transmission.

Yellow fever vaccine recommendation: no

Malaria: Malaria risk—predominantly due to *P. vivax*—exists throughout the year below 1500 m. There is moderate to high risk in the departments of Alta Verapaz, Baja Verapaz, Escuintla, Huehuetenango, Izabal, Petén, Quiché (Ixcan) and Retalhuleu.

Recommended prevention in risk areas: **II**

GUINEA

Yellow fever:

Country requirement: A yellow fever vaccination certificate is required from travellers over 1 year of age coming from areas with risk of yellow fever transmission.

Yellow fever vaccine recommendation: yes

Malaria: Malaria risk—predominantly due to *P. falciparum*—exists throughout the year in the whole country. Resistance to chloroquine reported.

Recommended prevention: **IV**

GUINEA-BISSAU

Yellow fever:

Country requirement: A yellow fever vaccination certificate is required from travellers over 1 year of age coming from areas with risk of yellow fever transmission, and from the following countries:

Africa: Angola, Benin, Burkina Faso, Burundi, Cape Verde, Central African Republic, Chad, Congo, Côte d'Ivoire, Democratic Republic of the Congo, Djibouti, Equatorial Guinea, Ethiopia, Gabon, Gambia, Ghana, Guinea, Kenya, Liberia, Madagascar, Mali, Mauritania, Mozambique, Niger, Nigeria, Rwanda, Sao Tome and Principe, Senegal, Sierra Leone, Somalia, Togo, Uganda, United Republic of Tanzania, Zambia.

America: Bolivia, Brazil, Colombia, Ecuador, French Guiana, Guyana, Panama, Peru, Suriname, Venezuela.

Yellow fever vaccine recommendation: yes

Malaria: Malaria risk—predominantly due to *P. falciparum*—exists throughout the year in the whole country. Resistance to chloroquine and sulfadoxine—pyrimethamine reported.

Recommended prevention: **IV**

GUYANA

Yellow fever:

Country requirement: A yellow fever vaccination certificate is required from travellers coming from areas with risk of yellow fever transmission and from the following countries:

Africa: Angola, Benin, Burkina Faso, Burundi, Cameroon, Central African Republic, Chad, Congo, Côte d'Ivoire, Democratic Republic of the Congo, Gabon, Gambia, Ghana, Guinea, Guinea-Bissau, Kenya, Liberia, Mali, Niger, Nigeria, Rwanda, Sao Tome and Principe, Senegal, Sierra Leone, Somalia, Togo, Uganda, United Republic of Tanzania.

America: Belize, Bolivia, Brazil, Colombia, Costa Rica, Ecuador, French Guiana, Guatemala, Honduras, Nicaragua, Panama, Peru, Suriname, Venezuela.

Yellow fever vaccine recommendation: yes

Malaria: Malaria risk—*P. falciparum* (42–48%), *P. vivax* (52–58%)—is high throughout the year in all parts of the interior. Highest risk occurs in Regions 1, 7, 8 and 9; moderate risk in Region 2; and low risk in Regions 4, 6 and 10. Sporadic cases of malaria have been reported from the densely populated coastal belt. Chloroquine-resistant *P. falciparum* reported.

Recommended prevention in risk areas: **IV**

HAITI

Yellow fever:

Country requirement: A yellow fever vaccination certificate is required from travellers coming from areas with risk of yellow fever transmission.

Yellow fever vaccine recommendation: no

Malaria: Malaria risk—exclusively due to *P. falciparum*—exists throughout the year in certain forest areas in Chantal, Gros Morne, Hinche, Jacmel and Maissade. In the other cantons, risk is estimated to be low. No *P. falciparum* resistance to chloroquine reported.

Recommended prevention in risk areas: **II**

HONDURAS

Yellow fever:

Country requirement: A yellow fever vaccination certificate is required from travellers coming from areas with risk of yellow fever transmission.

Yellow fever vaccine recommendation: no

Malaria: Malaria risk—predominantly due to *P. vivax*—is high throughout the year in the provinces of Colón, Gracias a Dios, and Islas de la Bahía; and moderate in the province of Atlántida. *P. falciparum* risk is the highest in Colón, Gracias a Dios, and the Islas de la Bahía.

Recommended prevention: **II**

HONG KONG SPECIAL ADMINISTRATIVE REGION OF CHINA *see* CHINA

HUNGARY

Yellow fever:

Country requirement: no

Yellow fever vaccine recommendation: no

ICELAND

Yellow fever:

Country requirement: no

Yellow fever vaccine recommendation: no

INDIA

Yellow fever:

Country requirement: Anyone (except infants up to the age of 6 months) arriving by air or sea without a certificate is detained in isolation for up to 6 days if that person (i) arrives within 6 days of departure from an area with risk of yellow fever transmission, or (ii) has been in such an area in transit (excepting those passengers and members of the crew who, while in transit through an airport situated in an area with risk of yellow fever transmission, remained within the airport premises during the period of their entire stay and the Health Officer agrees to such exemption), or (iii) has come on a ship that started from or touched at any port in a yellow fever area with risk of yellow fever transmission up to 30 days before its arrival in India, unless such a ship has been disinsected in accordance with the procedure laid down by WHO, or (iv) has come by an aircraft which has been in an area with risk of yellow fever transmission and has not been disinsected in accordance with the provisions laid down in the Indian Aircraft Public Health Rules, 1954, or those recommended by WHO. The following countries and areas are regarded as risk of yellow fever transmission:

Africa: Angola, Benin, Burkina Faso, Burundi, Cameroon, Central African Republic, Chad, Congo, Côte d'Ivoire, Democratic Republic of the Congo, Equatorial Guinea, Ethiopia, Gabon, Gambia, Ghana, Guinea, Guinea-Bissau, Kenya, Liberia, Mali, Niger, Nigeria, Rwanda, Sao Tome and Principe, Senegal, Sierra Leone, Somalia, Sudan, Togo, Uganda, United Republic of Tanzania, Zambia.

America: Bolivia, Brazil, Colombia, Ecuador, French Guiana, Guyana, Panama, Peru, Suriname, Trinidad and Tobago, Venezuela.

Note. When a case of yellow fever is reported from any country, that country is regarded by the Government of India as a country with risk of yellow fever and is added to the above list.

Yellow fever vaccine recommendations for travellers: no

Malaria: Malaria risk exists throughout the year in the whole country below 2000 m, with overall 40% to 50% of cases due to *P. falciparum*. There is no transmission in parts of the states of Himachal Pradesh, Jammu and Kashmir, and Sikkim. Risk of falciparum malaria and drug resistance are relatively higher in the north-eastern states, in Andaman and Nicobar Islands, Chhattisgarh, Goa, Gujarat, Jharkhand, Karnataka (with exception of the city of Bangalore), Madhya Pradesh, Maharashtra (with the exception of the cities of Mumbai, Nagpur, Nasik and Pune), Orissa and West Bengal (with the exception of the city of Kolkata) *P. falciparum* resistance to chloroquine and sulfadoxine–pyrimethamine reported.

Recommended prevention: **III**. In the listed higher risk areas: **IV**.

INDONESIA

Yellow fever:

Country requirement: A yellow fever vaccination certificate is required from travellers coming from areas with risk of yellow fever transmission.

Yellow fever vaccine recommendation: no

Malaria: Malaria risk exists throughout the year in the whole country except in Jakarta Municipality, big cities, and within the areas of the tourist resorts of Bali and Java. *P. falciparum* resistant to chloroquine and sulfadoxine–pyrimethamine reported. *P. vivax* resistant to chloroquine reported.

Recommended prevention in risk areas: **IV**

IRAN, ISLAMIC REPUBLIC OF

Yellow fever:

Country requirement: A yellow fever vaccination certificate is required from travellers coming from areas with risk of yellow fever transmission.

Yellow fever vaccine recommendation: no

Malaria: Limited risk—exclusively due to *P. vivax*—exists during the summer months in Ardebil and East Azerbaijan provinces north of the Zagros mountains. Malaria risk due to *P. vivax* and *P. falciparum* exists from March through November in rural areas

of the provinces of Hormozgan, Kerman (tropical part) and the southern part of Sistan–Baluchestan. *P. falciparum* resistant to chloroquine and sulfadoxine–pyrimethamine reported.

Recommended prevention: **II** in *P. vivax* risk areas; **IV** in *P. falciparum* risk areas.

IRAQ

Yellow fever:

Country requirement: A yellow fever vaccination certificate is required from travellers coming from areas with risk of yellow fever transmission.

Yellow fever vaccine recommendation: no

Malaria: Malaria risk—exclusively due to *P. vivax*—exists from May through November, principally in areas in the north below 1500 m (Duhok, Erbil and Sulaimaniya provinces) but also in Basrah Province.

Recommended prevention: **II**

IRELAND

Yellow fever:

Country requirement: no

Yellow fever vaccine recommendation: no

ISRAEL

Yellow fever:

Country requirement: no

Yellow fever vaccine recommendation: no

ITALY

Yellow fever:

Country requirement: no

Yellow fever vaccine recommendation: no

JAMAICA

Yellow fever:

Country requirement: A yellow fever vaccination certificate is required from travellers over 1 year of age coming from areas with risk of yellow fever transmission.

Yellow fever vaccine recommendation: no

JAPAN

Yellow fever:

Country requirement: no

Yellow fever vaccine recommendation: no

JORDAN

Yellow fever:

Country requirement: A yellow fever vaccination certificate is required from travellers over 1 year of age coming from areas with risk of yellow fever transmission.

Yellow fever vaccine recommendation: no

KAZAKHSTAN

Yellow fever:

Country requirement: A yellow fever vaccination certificate is required from travellers coming from areas with risk of yellow fever transmission.

Yellow fever vaccine recommendation: no

KENYA

Yellow fever:

Country requirement: A yellow fever vaccination certificate is required from travellers over 1 year of age coming from areas with risk of yellow fever transmission.

Yellow fever vaccine recommendation: yes (low risk in cities of Nairobi and Mombasa)

Malaria: Malaria risk—predominantly due to *P. falciparum*—exists throughout the year in the whole country. There is normally little risk in the city of Nairobi and in the highlands (above 2500 m) of Central, Eastern, Nyanza, Rift Valley and Western provinces. Resistance to chloroquine and sulfadoxine–pyrimethamine reported.

Recommended prevention: **IV**

KIRIBATI

Yellow fever:

Country requirement: A yellow fever vaccination certificate is required from travellers over 1 year of age coming from areas with risk of yellow fever transmission.

Yellow fever vaccine recommendation: no

KOREA, DEMOCRATIC PEOPLE'S REPUBLIC OF

Yellow fever:

Country requirement: no

Yellow fever vaccine recommendation: no

Malaria: Limited malaria risk—exclusively due to *P. vivax*—exists in some southern areas.

Recommended prevention: **I**

KOREA, REPUBLIC OF

Yellow fever:

Country requirement: no

Yellow fever vaccine recommendation: no

Malaria: Limited malaria risk—exclusively due to *P. vivax*—exists mainly in the northern areas of Kyunggi Do and Gangwon Do Provinces.

Recommended prevention: **I**

KUWAIT

Yellow fever:

Country requirement: no

Yellow fever vaccine recommendation: no

KYRGYZSTAN

Yellow fever:

Country requirement: no

Yellow fever vaccine recommendation: no

Malaria: Malaria risk – exclusively due to *P. vivax* – exists from June through October in some southern and western parts of the country, mainly in areas bordering Tajikistan and Uzbekistan – Batken, Osh and Jalal-Abad regions. The first case of autochtonous *P. falciparum* malaria was reported in 2004 in the southern part of the country, in an area bordering Uzbekistan.

Recommended prevention: **I**

LAO PEOPLE'S DEMOCRATIC REPUBLIC

Yellow fever:

Country requirement: A yellow fever vaccination certificate is required from travellers coming from areas with risk of yellow fever transmission.

Yellow fever vaccine recommendation: no

Malaria: Malaria risk—predominantly due to *P. falciparum*—exists throughout the year in the whole country except in Vientiane. Chloroquine and sulfadoxine–pyrimethamine resistant *P. falciparum* reported.

Recommended prevention: **IV**

LATVIA

Yellow fever:

Country requirement: no

Yellow fever vaccine recommendation: no

LEBANON

Yellow fever:

Country requirement: A yellow fever vaccination certificate is required from travellers coming from areas with risk of yellow fever transmission.

Yellow fever vaccine recommendation: no

LESOTHO

Yellow fever:

Country requirement: A yellow fever vaccination certificate is required from travellers coming from areas with risk of yellow fever transmission.

Yellow fever vaccine recommendation: no

LIBERIA

Yellow fever:

Country requirement: A yellow fever vaccination certificate is required from all travellers over year of age.

Yellow fever vaccine recommendation: yes

Malaria: Malaria risk—predominantly due to *P. falciparum*—exists throughout the year in the whole country. Resistance to chloroquine and sulfadoxine–pyrimethamine reported.

Recommended prevention: **IV**

LIBYAN ARAB JAMAHIRIYA

Yellow fever:

Country requirement: A yellow fever vaccination certificate is required from travellers coming from areas with risk of yellow fever transmission.

Yellow fever vaccine recommendation: no

LIECHTENSTEIN

Yellow fever:

Country requirement: no

Yellow fever vaccine recommendation: no

LITHUANIA

Yellow fever:

Country requirement: no

Yellow fever vaccine recommendation: no

LUXEMBOURG

Yellow fever:

Country requirement: no

Yellow fever vaccine recommendation: no

MACAO SPECIAL ADMINISTRATIVE REGION OF CHINA SEE CHINA

MACEDONIA, THE FORMER YUGOSLAV REPUBLIC OF

Yellow fever:

Country requirement: no

Yellow fever vaccine recommendation: no

MADAGASCAR

Yellow fever:

Country requirement: A yellow fever vaccination certificate is required from travellers coming from areas with risk of yellow fever transmission.

Yellow fever vaccine recommendation: no

Malaria: Malaria risk—predominantly due to *P. falciparum*—exists throughout the year in the whole country, with the highest risk in the coastal areas. Resistance to chloroquine reported.

Recommended prevention: **IV**

MADEIRA ISLANDS *see* PORTUGAL

MALAWI

Yellow fever:

Country requirement: A yellow fever vaccination certificate is required from travellers coming from areas with risk of yellow fever transmission.

Yellow fever vaccine recommendation: no

Malaria: Malaria risk—predominantly due to *P. falciparum*—exists throughout the year in the whole country. Resistance to chloroquine and sulfadoxine–pyrimethamine reported.

Recommended prevention: **IV**

MALAYSIA

Yellow fever:

Country requirement: A yellow fever vaccination certificate is required from travellers over 1 year of age arriving within 6 days from areas with risk of yellow fever transmission.

Yellow fever vaccine recommendation: no

Malaria: Malaria risk exists only in limited foci in the deep hinterland. Urban and coastal areas are free from malaria. *P. falciparum* resistant to chloroquine and sulfadoxine–pyrimethamine reported.

Recommended prevention in risk areas: **IV**

MALDIVES

Yellow fever:

Country requirement: A yellow fever vaccination certificate is required from travellers coming from areas with risk of yellow fever transmission.

Yellow fever vaccine recommendation: no

MALI

Yellow fever:

Country requirement: A yellow fever vaccination certificate is required from all travellers over 1 year of age.

Yellow fever vaccine recommendation: yes

Malaria: Malaria risk—predominantly due to *P. falciparum*—exists throughout the year in the whole country. Resistance to chloroquine and sulfadoxine–pyrimethamine reported.

Recommended prevention: **IV**

MALTA

Yellow fever:

Country requirement: A yellow fever vaccination certificate is required from travellers over 9 months of age coming from areas with risk of yellow fever transmission. If indicated on epidemiological grounds, infants under 9 months of age are subject to isolation or surveillance if coming from an area with risk of yellow fever transmission.

Yellow fever vaccine recommendation: no

MARSHALL ISLANDS

Yellow fever:

Country requirement: no

Yellow fever vaccine recommendation: no

MARTINIQUE

Yellow fever:

Country requirement: no

Yellow fever vaccine recommendation: no

MAURITANIA

Yellow fever:

Country requirement: A yellow fever vaccination certificate is required from all travellers over 1 year of age, except those coming from an area without a risk of yellow fever transmission and staying less than 2 weeks in the country.

Yellow fever vaccine recommendation: yes

Malaria: Malaria risk—predominantly due to *P. falciparum*—exists throughout the year in the whole country, except in the northern areas: Dakhlet-Nouadhibou and Tiris-Zemour. In Adrar and Inchiri there is malaria risk during the rainy season (July through October). Resistance to chloroquine reported.

Recommended prevention in risk areas: **IV**

MAURITIUS

Yellow fever:

Country requirement: A yellow fever vaccination certificate is required from travellers over 1 year of age coming from areas with risk of yellow fever transmission.

Yellow fever vaccine recommendation: no

Malaria: Malaria risk—exclusively due to *P. vivax*—may exist in certain rural areas (no indigenous cases reported since 1998). There is no risk on Rodrigues Island.

Recommended prevention: **none**

MAYOTTE (FRENCH TERRITORIAL COLLECTIVITY)

Yellow fever:

Country requirement: no

Yellow fever vaccine recommendation: no

Malaria: Malaria risk—predominantly due to *P. falciparum*—exists throughout the year. Resistance to chloroquine and sulfadoxine–pyrimethamine reported.

Recommended prevention: **IV**

MEXICO

Yellow fever:

Country requirement: no

Yellow fever vaccine recommendation: no

Malaria: Malaria risk—almost exclusively due to *P. vivax*—exists throughout the year in some rural areas that are not often visited by tourists. There is high risk of transmission in some localities in the states of Chiapas and Oaxaca; moderate risk in the states of Chihuahua, Sinaloa and Tabasco; and low risk in Campeche, Durango, Guerrero, Michoacán, Jalisco, Nayarit, Quintana Roo, Sonora, Veracruz and Yucatan.

Recommended prevention in risk areas: **II**

MICRONESIA, FEDERATED STATES OF

Yellow fever:

Country requirement: no

Yellow fever vaccine recommendation: no

MOLDOVA, REPUBLIC OF

Yellow fever:

Country requirement: no

Yellow fever vaccine recommendation: no

MONACO

Yellow fever:

Country requirement: no

Yellow fever vaccine recommendation: no

MONGOLIA

Yellow fever:

Country requirement: no

Yellow fever vaccine recommendation: no

MONTENEGRO

Yellow fever:

Country requirement: no

Yellow fever vaccine recommendation: no

MONTSERRAT

Yellow fever:

Country requirement: A yellow fever vaccination certificate is required from travellers over 1 year of age coming from areas with risk of yellow fever transmission.

Yellow fever vaccine recommendation: no

MOROCCO

Yellow fever:

Country requirement: no

Yellow fever vaccine recommendation: no

Malaria: Very limited malaria risk—exclusively due to *P. vivax*—may exist from May to October in certain rural areas of Chefchaouen Province (no indigenous cases reported in 2005).

Recommended prevention: **I**

MOZAMBIQUE

Yellow fever:

Country requirement: A yellow fever vaccination certificate is required from travellers over 1 year of age coming from areas with risk of yellow fever transmission.

Yellow fever vaccine recommendation: no

Malaria: Malaria risk—predominantly due to *P. falciparum*—exists throughout the year in the whole country. Resistance to chloroquine and sulfadoxine–pyrimethamine reported.

Recommended prevention: **IV**

MYANMAR (FORMERLY BURMA)

Yellow fever:

Country requirement: A yellow fever vaccination certificate is required from travellers coming from areas with risk of yellow fever transmission. Nationals and residents of Myanmar are required to possess certificates of vaccination on their departure to an area with risk of yellow fever transmission.

Yellow fever vaccine recommendation: no

Malaria: Malaria risk—predominantly due to *P. falciparum*—exists throughout the year at altitudes below 1000 m, excluding the main urban areas of Yangon and Mandalay. Risk is highest in remote rural, hilly and forested areas. *P. falciparum* resistant to chloroquine and sulfadoxine–pyrimethamine reported. Mefloquine resistance reported in Kayin state and the eastern part of Shan state. *P. vivax* with reduced sensitivity to chloroquine reported.

Recommended prevention: **IV**

NAMIBIA

Yellow fever:

Country requirement: A yellow fever vaccination certificate is required from travellers coming from areas with risk of yellow fever transmission. The countries, or parts of countries, included in the endemic zones in Africa and South America are regarded as risk of yellow fever transmission. Travellers on scheduled flights that originated outside the areas with risk of yellow fever transmission, but who have been in transit through these areas, are not required to possess a certificate provided that they remained at the scheduled airport or in the adjacent town during transit. All passengers whose flights originated in areas with risk of yellow fever transmission or who have been in transit through these areas on unscheduled flights are required to possess a certificate. The certificate is not insisted upon in the case of children under

1 year of age, but such infants may be subject to surveillance.

Yellow fever vaccine recommendation: no

Malaria: Malaria risk—predominantly due to *P. falciparum*—exists from November to June in the following regions: Oshana, Oshikoto, Omusati, Omaheke, Ohangwena and Otjozondjupa. Risk throughout the year exists along the Kunene river and in Kavango and Caprivi regions. Resistance to chloroquine and sulfadoxine–pyrimethamine reported.

Recommended prevention in risk areas: **IV**

NAURU
Yellow fever:

Country requirement: A yellow fever vaccination certificate is required from travellers over 1 year of age coming from areas with risk of yellow fever transmission.

Yellow fever vaccine recommendation: no

NEPAL
Yellow fever:

Country requirement: A yellow fever vaccination certificate is required from travellers coming from areas with risk of yellow fever transmission.

Yellow fever vaccine recommendation: no

Malaria: Malaria risk—predominantly due to *P. vivax*—exists throughout the year in rural areas of the 20 Terai districts (including forested hills and forest areas) bordering with India, and in parts of the inner Terai valleys of Udaypur, Sindhupalchowk, Makwanpur, Chitwan and Dang. *P. falciparum* resistant to chloroquine and sulfadoxine–pyrimethamine reported.

Recommended prevention in risk areas: **III**

NETHERLANDS
Yellow fever:

Country requirement: no

Yellow fever vaccine recommendation: no

NETHERLANDS ANTILLES
Yellow fever:

Country requirement: A yellow fever vaccination certificate is required from travellers over 6 months

of age coming from area with risk of yellow fever transmission.

Yellow fever vaccine recommendation: no

NEW CALEDONIA AND DEPENDENCIES
Yellow fever:

Country requirement: A yellow fever vaccination certificate is required from travellers over 1 year of age coming from areas with risk of yellow fever transmission.

Note. In the event of an epidemic threat to the territory, a specific vaccination certificate may be required.

Yellow fever vaccine recommendation: no

NEW ZEALAND
Yellow fever:

Country requirement: no

Yellow fever vaccine recommendation: no

NICARAGUA
Yellow fever:

Country requirement: A yellow fever vaccination certificate is required from travellers over 1 year of age coming from areas with risk of yellow fever transmission.

Yellow fever vaccine recommendation: no

Malaria: Malaria risk—predominantly due to *P. vivax*—exists throughout the year in 119 munic-ipalities, with the highest risk in 7 municipalities in the department of RA Atlántico Sur and moderate risk in 6 municipalites in RA Atlántico Norte. Cases are reported from 138 other municipalities in the central and western department; but the risk in these areas is considered low or negligible. No chloroquine-resistant P. falciparum reported.

Recommended prevention in risk areas: **II**

NIGER
Yellow fever:

Country requirement: A yellow fever vaccination certificate is required from all travellers over 1 year of age and recommended for travellers leaving Niger.

Malaria: Malaria risk—predominantly due to *P. falciparum*—exists throughout the year in the whole country. Chloroquine-resistant *P. falciparum* reported.

Recommended prevention: **IV**

NIGERIA

Yellow fever:

Country requirement: A yellow fever vaccination certificate is required from travellers over 1 year of age coming from areas with risk of yellow fever transmission.

Yellow fever vaccine recommendation: yes

Malaria: Malaria risk—predominantly due to *P. falciparum*—exists throughout the year in the whole country. Resistance to chloroquine and sulfadoxine–pyrimethamine reported.

Recommended prevention: **IV**

NIUE

Yellow fever:

Country requirement: A yellow fever vaccination certificate is required from travellers over 1 year of age coming from areas with risk of yellow fever transmission.

Yellow fever vaccine recommendation: no

NORFOLK ISLAND *see* AUSTRALIA

NORTHERN MARIANA ISLANDS

Yellow fever:

Country requirement: no

Yellow fever vaccine recommendation: no

NORWAY

Yellow fever:

Country requirement: no

Yellow fever vaccine recommendation: no

OMAN

Yellow fever:

Country requirement: A yellow fever vaccination certificate is required from travellers coming from areas with risk of yellow fever transmission.

Yellow fever vaccine recommendation: no

Malaria: No indigenous *P. vivax* or *P. falciparum* cases reported since 2001.

Recommended prevention: **none**

PAKISTAN

Yellow fever:

Country requirement: A yellow fever vaccination certificate is required from travellers coming from any part of a country in which there is a risk of yellow fever transmission; infants under 6 months of age are exempt if the mother's vaccination certificate shows that she was vaccinated before the birth of the child.

Yellow fever vaccine recommendation: no

Malaria: Malaria risk—*P. vivax* and *P. falciparum*—exists throughout the year in the whole country below 2000 m. *P. falciparum* resistant to chloroquine and sulfadoxine–pyrimethamine reported.

Recommended prevention: **IV**

PALAU

Yellow fever:

Country requirement: A yellow fever vaccination certificate is required from all travellers over 1 year of age coming from countries with risk of yellow fever transmission or from countries in any part of which there is a risk of yellow fever transmission.

Yellow fever vaccine recommendation: no

PANAMA

Yellow fever:

Country requirement: A yellow fever vaccination certificate is required from all travellers coming from countries with risk of yellow fever transmission

Yellow fever vaccination recommendation: recommended for all travellers who are going to the Province of Darien, the region Kuna Yala (old San Blas), East Panama including the districts of Chep, Chiman and Balboa. This does not include the City of Panama and the Panama Canal area (old Canal Zone).

Malaria: Malaria risk—predominantly due to *P. vivax* (83%); *P. falciparum* (17%)—exists throughout the year in provinces along the Atlantic coast and the border with Colombia: Bocas del Toro, Colon, Darien, Embera, Kuna Yala, Ngobe Bugle, Panama and Veraguas. In Panama City, the Canal zone, and in the other provinces there is no or negligible risk of transmission.

Chloroquine-resistant *P. falciparum* has been reported in Darién and San Blas provinces.

Recommended prevention in risk areas: **II**; in eastern endemic areas, **IV**

PAPUA NEW GUINEA

Yellow fever:

Country requirement: A yellow fever vaccination certificate is required from all travellers over 1 year of age coming from areas with risk of yellow fever transmission.

Yellow fever vaccine recommendation: no

Malaria: Malaria risk—predominantly due to *P. falciparum*—exists throughout the year in the whole country below 1800 m. *P. falciparum* resistant to chloroquine and sulfadoxine–pyrimethamine reported. *P. vivax* resistant to chloroquine reported.

Recommended prevention: **IV**

PARAGUAY

Yellow fever:

Country requirement: A yellow fever vaccination certificate is required from travellers coming from areas with risk of yellow fever transmission.

Yellow fever vaccine recommendation: No. Vaccination is recommended for travellers visiting Iguaçu Falls

Malaria: Malaria risk—exclusively due to *P. vivax*—is moderate in certain municipalities of the departments of Alto Paraná, Caaguazú, Caazapa, Canendiyú and Guaira. In the other departments there is no or negligible transmission risk.

Recommended prevention in risk areas: **II**

PERU

Yellow fever:

Country requirement: no

Yellow fever recommendation: recommended for those who intend to visit the jungle areas of the country below 2300m. Travellers who will only visit the cities of Cuzco and Machu Picchu do not need vaccination.

Malaria: Malaria risk—*P. vivax* (84%), *P. falciparum* (16%)—is high in 21 of the 33 sanitary regions, including Ayacucho, Cajamarca, Cerro de Pasco, Chachapoyas, Chanca-Andahuaylas, Cutervo, Cusco, Huancavelica, Jaen, Junín, La Libertad, Lambayeque, Loreto, Madre de Dios, Piura, San Martín, Tumbes and Ucayali. *P. falciparum* transmission reported in Jaen, Lambayeque, Loreto, Luciano Castillo, Piura, San Martín, Tumbes and Ucayali. Resistance to chloroquine and sulfadoxine–pyrimethamine reported.

Recommended prevention: **II** in *P. vivax* risk areas; **IV** in *P. falciparum* risk areas.

PHILIPPINES

Yellow fever:

Country requirement: A yellow fever vaccination certificate is required from travellers over 1 year of age coming from areas with risk of yellow fever transmission.

Yellow fever vaccine recommendation: no

Malaria: Malaria risk exists throughout the year in areas below 600 m, except in the provinces of Aklan, Benguet, Bilaran, Bohol, Camiguin, Capiz, Catanduanes, Cebu, Guimaras, Iloilo, Leyte, Masbate, northern Samar, Sequijor and metropolitan Manila. No risk is considered to exist in urban areas or in the plains. *P. falciparum* resistant to chloroquine and sulfadoxine–pyrimethamine reported.

Recommended prevention in risk areas: **IV**

PITCAIRN

Yellow fever:

Country requirement: A yellow fever vaccination certificate is required from travellers over 1 year of age coming from areas with risk of yellow fever transmission.

Yellow fever vaccine recommendation: no

POLAND

Yellow fever:

Country requirement: no

Yellow fever vaccine recommendation: no

PORTUGAL

Yellow fever:

Country requirement: A yellow fever vaccination certificate is required from travellers over 1 year of age coming from areas with risk of yellow fever transmission. The requirement applies only to travellers arriving in or bound for the Azores and Madeira. However, no certificate is required from passengers in transit at Funchal, Porto Santo and Santa Maria.

Yellow fever vaccine recommendation: no

PUERTO RICO

Yellow fever:

Country requirement: no

Yellow fever vaccine recommendation: no

QATAR

Yellow fever:

Country requirement: no

Yellow fever vaccine recommendation: no

REPUBLIC OF KOREA *see* KOREA, REPUBLIC OF

REPUBLIC OF MOLDOVA *see* MOLDOVA, REPUBLIC OF

REUNION

Yellow fever:

Country requirement: A yellow fever vaccination certificate is required from travellers over 1 year of age coming from areas with risk of yellow fever transmission.

Yellow fever vaccine recommendation: no

ROMANIA

Yellow fever:

Country requirement: no

Yellow fever vaccine recommendation: no

RUSSIAN FEDERATION

Yellow fever:

Country requirement: no

Yellow fever vaccine recommendation: no

RWANDA

Yellow fever:

Country requirement: A yellow fever vaccination certificate is required from all travellers over 1 year of age.

Malaria: Malaria risk—predominantly due to *P. falciparum*—exists throughout the year in the whole country. Resistance to chloroquine and sulfadoxine–pyrimethamine reported.

Recommended prevention: **IV**

SAINT HELENA

Yellow fever:

Country requirement: A yellow fever vaccination certificate is required from travellers over 1 year of age coming from areas with risk of yellow fever transmission.

Yellow fever vaccine recommendation: no

SAINT KITTS AND NEVIS

Yellow fever:

Country requirement: A yellow fever vaccination certificate is required from travellers over 1 year of age coming from areas with risk of yellow fever transmission.

Yellow fever vaccine recommendation: no

SAINT LUCIA

Yellow fever:

Country requirement: A yellow fever vaccination certificate is required from travellers over 1 year of age coming from areas with risk of yellow fever transmission.

Yellow fever vaccine recommendation: no

SAINT PIERRE AND MIQUELON

Yellow fever:

Country requirement: no

Yellow fever vaccine recommendation: no

SAINT VINCENT AND THE GRENADINES

Yellow fever:

Country requirement: A yellow fever vaccination certificate is required from travellers over 1 year of age coming from areas with risk of yellow fever transmission.

Yellow fever vaccine recommendation: no

SAMOA

Yellow fever:

Country requirement: A yellow fever vaccination certificate is required from travellers over 1 year of age coming from areas with risk of yellow fever transmission.

Yellow fever vaccine recommendation: no

SAN MARINO

Yellow fever:

Country requirement: no

Yellow fever vaccine recommendation: no

SAO TOME AND PRINCIPE

Yellow fever:

Country requirement: A yellow fever vaccination certificate is required from travellers over 1 year of age.

Malaria: Malaria risk—predominantly due to *P. falciparum*—exists throughout the year. Chloroquine-resistant *P. falciparum* reported.

Recommended prevention: **IV**

SAUDI ARABIA

Yellow fever:

Country requirement: A yellow fever vaccination certificate is required from all travellers coming from countries with risk of yellow fever transmission.

Yellow fever vaccine recommendation: no

Malaria: Malaria risk—predominantly due to *P. falciparum*—exists throughout the year in most of the South-western Region (except in the high-altitude areas of Asir Province). No risk in Mecca or Medina cities. Chloroquine-resistant *P. falciparum* reported.

Recommended prevention in risk areas: **IV**

SENEGAL

Yellow fever:

Country requirement: A yellow fever vaccination certificate is required from travellers coming from areas with risk of yellow fever transmission.

Yellow fever vaccine recommendation: yes

Malaria: Malaria risk—predominantly due to *P. falciparum*—exists throughout the year in the whole country. There is less risk from January through June in the central western regions. Resistance to chloroquine and sulfadoxine–pyrimethamine reported.

Recommended prevention: **IV**

SERBIA

Yellow fever:

Country requirement: no

Yellow fever vaccine recommendation: no

SEYCHELLES

Yellow fever:

Country requirement: A yellow fever vaccination certificate is required from travellers over 1 year of age coming from areas with risk of yellow fever transmission within the preceding 6 days.

Yellow fever vaccine recommendation: no

SIERRA LEONE

Yellow fever:

Country requirement: A yellow fever vaccination certificate is required from all travellers .

Malaria: Malaria risk—predominantly due to *P. falciparum*—exists throughout the year in the whole country. Resistance to chloroquine and sulfadoxine–pyrimethamine reported.

Recommended prevention: **IV**

SINGAPORE

Yellow fever:

Country requirement: Certificates of vaccination are required from travellers over 1 year of age who, within the preceding 6 days, have been in or have passed through any country partly or wholly endemic for yellow fever. The countries and areas included in the endemic zones are considered as areas with risk of yellow fever transmission:

Africa: Angola, Benin, Burkina Faso, Burundi, Cameroon, Cape Verde, Central African Republic, Chad, Congo, Cote d'Ivoire, Democratic Republic of Congo, Equatorial Guinea, Ethiopia, Gabon, Gambia, Ghana, Guinea, Guinea–Bissau, Kenya, Liberia,, Mali, Mauritania, Niger, Nigeria, Rwanda, Sao Tome and Principe, Senegal, Sierra Leone, Somalia, Sudan, Togo, Uganda, United Republic of Tanzania.

America: Argentina, Bolivia, Brazil, Colombia, Ecuador, French Guyana, Guyana, Panama, Paraguay, Peru, Trinidad and Tobago, Suriname, Venezuela.

Yellow fever vaccine recommendation for travellers: no

SLOVAKIA

Yellow fever:

Country requirement: no

Yellow fever vaccine recommendation: no

SLOVENIA

Yellow fever:

Country requirement: no

Yellow fever vaccine recommendation: no

SOLOMON ISLANDS

Yellow fever:

Country requirement: A yellow fever vaccination certificate is required from travellers coming from areas with risk of yellow fever transmission.

Yellow fever vaccine recommendation: no

Malaria: Malaria risk—predominantly due to *P. falciparum*—exists throughout the year except in a few eastern and southern outlying islets. *P. falciparum* resistant to chloroquine and sulfadoxine–pyrimethamine reported.

Recommended prevention: **IV**

SOMALIA

Yellow fever:

Country requirement: A yellow fever vaccination certificate is required from travellers coming from areas with risk of yellow fever transmission.

Yellow fever vaccine recommendation: yes

Malaria: Malaria risk—predominantly due to *P. falciparum*—exists throughout the year in the whole country. Resistance to chloroquine and sulfadoxine–pyrimethamine reported.

Recommended prevention: **IV**

SOUTH AFRICA

Yellow fever:

Country requirement: A yellow fever vaccination certificate is required from travellers over 1 year of age coming from areas with risk of yellow fever transmission.

Yellow fever vaccine recommendation: no

Malaria: Malaria risk—predominantly due to *P. falciparum*—exists throughout the year in the low altitude areas of Mpumalanga Province (including the Kruger National Park), Northern Province and north-eastern KwaZulu-Natal as far

south as the Tugela River. Risk is highest from October to May. Resistance to chloroquine and sulfadoxine–pyrimethamine reported.

Recommended prevention in risk areas: **IV**

SPAIN

Yellow fever:

Country requirement: no

Yellow fever vaccine recommendation: no

SRI LANKA

Yellow fever:

Country requirement: A yellow fever vaccination certificate is required from travellers over 1 year of age coming from areas with risk of yellow fever transmission.

Yellow fever vaccine recommendation: no

Malaria: Malaria risk—*P. vivax* (88%), *P. falciparum* (12%)—exists throughout the year, except in the districts of Colombo, Galle, Gampaha, Kalutara, Matara and Nuwara Eliya. *P. falciparum* resistant to chloroquine and sulfadoxine–pyrimethamine reported.

Recommended prevention in risk areas: **III**

SUDAN

Yellow fever:

Country requirement: A yellow fever vaccination certificate is required from travellers over 1 year of age coming from areas with risk of yellow fever transmission. A certificate may be required from travellers leaving Sudan.

Yellow fever vaccine recommendation: yes

Malaria: Malaria risk—predominantly due to *P. falciparum*—exists throughout the year in the whole country. Risk is low and seasonal in the north. It is higher along the Nile south of Lake Nasser and in the central and southern part of the country. Malaria risk on the Red Sea coast is very limited. Resistance to chloroquine and sulfadoxine–pyrimethamine reported.

Recommended prevention: **IV**

SURINAME

Yellow fever:

Country requirement: A yellow fever vaccination certificate is required from travellers coming from areas with risk of yellow fever transmission.

Yellow fever vaccine recommendation: yes

Malaria: Malaria risk—*P. falciparum* (81%)—is high throughout the year in the interior of the country beyond the coastal savannah area, with highest risk along the eastern border and in gold mining areas. In Paramaribo city and the other seven coastal districts, transmission risk is low or negligible. Chloroquine, sulfadoxine–pyrimethamine and mefloquine resistant *P. falciparum* reported. Some decline in quinine sensitivity also reported.

Recommended prevention in risk areas: **IV**

SWAZILAND

Yellow fever:

Country requirement: A yellow fever vaccination certificate is required from travellers coming from areas with risk of yellow fever transmission.

Yellow fever vaccine recommendation: no

Malaria: Malaria risk—predominantly due to *P. falciparum*—exists throughout the year in all low veld areas (mainly Big Bend, Mhlume, Simunye and Tshaneni). Chloroquine-resistant *P. falciparum* reported.

Recommended prevention in risk areas: **IV**

SWEDEN

Yellow fever:

Country requirement: no

Yellow fever vaccine recommendation: no

SWITZERLAND

Yellow fever:

Country requirement: no

Yellow fever vaccine recommendation: no

SYRIAN ARAB REPUBLIC

Yellow fever:

Country requirement: A yellow fever vaccination certificate is required from travellers coming from areas with risk of yellow fever transmission.

Yellow fever vaccine recommendation: no

Malaria: Limited malaria risk—exclusively due to *P. vivax*—exists from May through October in foci along the northern border, especially in rural areas of El Hasaka Governorate (no indigenous cases reported since 2005).

Recommended prevention in risk areas: **none**

TAJIKISTAN

Yellow fever:

Country requirement: no

Yellow fever vaccine recommendation: no

Malaria: Malaria risk—predominantly due to *P. vivax*—exists from June through October, particularly in southern border areas (Khatlon Region), and in some central (Dushanbe), western (Gorno-Badakhshan), and northern (Leninabad Region) areas. Chloroquine and sulfadoxine–pyrimethamine resistant *P. falciparum* reported in the southern part of the country.

Recommended prevention in risk areas: **III**

TANZANIA, UNITED REPUBLIC OF

Yellow fever:

Country requirement: A yellow fever vaccination certificate is required from travellers over 1 year of age coming from areas with risk of yellow fever transmission.

Yellow fever vaccine recommendation: yes

Malaria: Malaria risk—predominantly due to *P. falciparum*—exists throughout the year in the whole country below 1800 m. Resistance to chloroquine and sulfadoxine–pyrimethamine reported.

Recommended prevention: **IV**

THAILAND

Yellow fever:

Country requirement: A yellow fever vaccination certificate is required from travellers over 1 year of age coming from areas with risk of yellow fever transmission.

Yellow fever vaccine recommendation: no

Malaria: Malaria risk exists throughout the year in rural, especially forested and hilly, areas of the whole country, mainly towards the international borders. There is no risk in cities (e.g. Bangkok, Chiangmai city, Pattaya), Samui island and the main tourist resorts of Phuket island. However, there is a risk in some other areas and islands. *P. falciparum* resistant to chloroquine and sulfadoxine–pyrimethamine reported. Resistance to mefloquine and to quinine reported from areas near the borders with Cambodia and Myanmar.

Recommended prevention in risk areas: **I**; in areas near Cambodia and Myanmar borders: **IV**

TIMOR LESTE

Yellow Fever:

Country requirement: A yellow fever vaccination certificate is required from travellers over 1 year of age coming from areas with risk of yellow fever transmission.

Yellow fever vaccine recommendation: no

Malaria: Malaria risk—predominantly due to *P. falciparum*—exists throughout the year in the whole territory. *P. falciparum* resistant to chloroquine and sulfadoxine–pyrimethamine reported.

Recommended prevention: **IV**

TOGO

Yellow fever:

Country requirement: A yellow fever vaccination certificate is required from all travellers over 1 year of age.

Malaria: Malaria risk—predominantly due to *P. falciparum*—exists throughout the year in the whole country. Chloroquine-resistant *P. falciparum* reported.

Recommended prevention: **IV**

TOKELAU

Same requirements as New Zealand.

(Non-self governing territory of New Zealand)

TONGA

Yellow fever:

Country requirement: A yellow fever vaccination certificate is required from travellers over 1 year of age coming from areas with risk of yellow fever transmission.

Yellow fever vaccine recommendation: no

TRINIDAD AND TOBAGO

Yellow fever:

Country requirement: A yellow fever vaccination certificate is required from travellers over 1 year of age coming from areas with risk of yellow fever transmission.

Yellow fever vaccine recommendation: yes

TUNISIA

Yellow fever:

Country requirement: A yellow fever vaccination certificate is required from travellers over 1 year of age coming from areas with risk of yellow fever transmission.

Yellow fever vaccine recommendation: no

TURKEY

Yellow fever:

Country requirement: no

Yellow fever vaccine recommendation: no

Malaria: Malaria risk—exclusively due to *P. vivax*—exists from May to October mainly in the south-eastern part of the country, and in Amikova and Çukurova Plain. There is no malaria risk in the main tourist areas in the west and south-west of the country.

Recommended prevention in risk areas: **II**

TURKMENISTAN

Yellow fever:

Country requirement: no

Yellow fever vaccine recommendation: no

Malaria: Malaria risk—exclusively due to *P. vivax*—exists from June to October in some villages located in the south-eastern part of the country, mainly in Mary district.

Recommended prevention: **I**

TUVALU

Yellow fever:

Country requirement: no

Yellow fever vaccine recommendation: no

UGANDA

Yellow fever:

Country requirement: A yellow fever vaccination certificate is required from travellers over 1 year of age coming from areas with risk of yellow fever transmission.

Yellow fever vaccine recommendation: yes

Malaria: Malaria risk—predominantly due to *P. falciparum*—exists throughout the year in the whole country including the main towns of Fort Portal, Jinja, Kampala, Mbale and parts of Kigezi.

Resistance to chloroquine and sulfadoxine–pyrimethamine reported.

Recommended prevention: **IV**

UKRAINE

Yellow fever:

Country requirement: no

Yellow fever vaccine recommendation: no

UNITED ARAB EMIRATES

Yellow fever:

Country requirement: no

Yellow fever vaccine recommendation: no

UNITED KINGDOM (WITH CHANNEL ISLANDS AND ISLE OF MAN)

Yellow fever:

Country requirement: no

Yellow fever vaccine recommendation: no

UNITED REPUBLIC OF TANZANIA see TANZANIA, UNITED REPUBLIC OF

UNITED STATES OF AMERICA

Yellow fever:

Country requirement: no

Yellow fever vaccine recommendation: no

URUGUAY

Yellow fever:

Country requirement: A yellow fever certificate is required for travellers coming from areas with risk of yellow fever transmission

Yellow fever vaccine recommendation: no

UZBEKISTAN

Yellow fever:

Country requirement: no

Yellow fever vaccine recommendation: no

Malaria: Sporadic autochthonous cases of *P. vivax* malaria are reported in some locations of Surkhanda-rinskaya Region.

Recommended prevention: **I**

VANUATU

Yellow fever:

Country requirement: no

Yellow fever vaccine recommendation: no

Malaria: Low to moderate malaria risk—predominantly due to *P. falciparum*—exists throughout the year in the whole country. *P. falciparum* resistant to chloroquine and sulfadoxine–pyrimethamine reported. *P. vivax* resistant to chloroquine reported.

Recommended prevention: **III**

VENEZUELA (BOLIVARIAN REPUBLIC OF)

Yellow fever:

Country requirement: no.

Yellow fever vaccine recommendation: yes

Malaria: Malaria risk—due to *P. vivax* (90%); *P. falciparum* (10%)—exists throughout the year in some rural areas of Apure, Amazonas, Barinas, Bolívar, Sucre and Táchira states. Risk of *P. falciparum* malaria is mostly restricted to municipalities in jungle areas of Amazonas (Alto Orinoco, Atabapo, Atures, Autana, Manapiare, Rio Negro), Bolívar (Cedeño, Gran Sabana, Piar, Raul Leoni, Sifontes and Sucre), Carabobo (Naguanagua) and Delta Amacuro (Antonia Diaz, Casacoima and Pedernales). Chloroquine and sulfadoxine–pyrimethamine resistant *P. falciparum* reported.

Recommended prevention: **II** in *P. vivax* risk areas; **IV** in *P. falciparum* risk areas.

VIET NAM

Yellow fever:

Country requirement: A yellow fever vaccination certificate is required from travellers over 1 year of age coming from areas with risk of yellow fever transmission.

Yellow fever vaccine recommendation: no

Malaria: Malaria risk—predominantly due to *P. falciparum*—exists in the whole country, excluding urban centres, the Red River delta, and the coastal plain areas of central Viet Nam. High-risk areas are the highland areas below 1500 m south of 18°N, notably in the 4 central highlands provinces Dak Lak, Dak Nong, Gia Lai and Kon Tum, Binh Phuoc province, and the western parts of the coastal provinces, Quang Tri, Quang Nam, Ninh Thuan and Khanh Hoa. Resistance to chloroquine, sulfadoxine–pyrimethamine and mefloquine reported.

Recommended prevention in risk areas: **IV**

VIRGIN ISLANDS (USA)

Yellow fever:

Country requirement: no

Yellow fever vaccine recommendation: no

WAKE ISLAND

Yellow fever:

Country requirement: no

Yellow fever vaccine recommendation: no

(US territory)

YEMEN

Yellow fever:

Country requirement: A yellow fever vaccination certificate is required from travellers over 1 year of age coming from areas with risk of yellow fever transmission.

Yellow fever vaccine recommendation: no

Malaria: Malaria risk—predominantly due to *P. falciparum*—exists throughout the year, but mainly from September through February, in the whole country below 2000 m. There is no risk in Sana'a city. Malaria risk on Socotra Island is limited. Resistance to chloroquine and sulfadoxine–pyrimethamine reported.

Recommended prevention in risk areas: **IV**; Socotra Island: **I**

ZAMBIA

Yellow fever:

Country requirement: no

Yellow fever vaccine recommendation: no

Malaria: Malaria risk—predominantly due to *P. falciparum*—exists throughout the year in the whole country. Resistance to chloroquine and sulfadoxine–pyrimethamine reported.

Recommended prevention: **IV**

ZIMBABWE

Yellow fever:

Country requirement: A yellow fever vaccination certificate is required from travellers coming from areas with risk of yellow fever transmission.

Yellow fever vaccine recommendation: no

Malaria: Malaria risk—predominantly due to *P. falciparum*—exists from November through June in areas below 1200 m and throughout the year in the Zambezi valley. In Harare and Bulawayo, the risk is negligible. Resistance to chloroquine and sulfadoxine–pyrimethamine reported.

Recommended prevention: **IV**

Countries with risk of yellow fever transmission* and countries requiring yellow fever vaccination

Countries	Countries with risk of yellow fever transmission*	Countries requiring yellow fever vaccination for travellers coming from countries with risk of yellow fever transmission*	Countries requiring yellow fever vaccination for travellers from all countries
Afghanistan		Yes	
Albania		Yes	
Algeria		Yes	
Angola	Yes		Yes
Anguilla		Yes	
Antigua and Barbuda		Yes	
Australia		Yes	
Bahamas		Yes	
Bangladesh		Yes	
Barbados		Yes	
Belize		Yes	
Benin	Yes		Yes
Bhutan		Yes	
Bolivia	Yes	Yes	

* Either yellow fever has been reported or disease in the past plus presence of vectors and animal reservoirs create a potential risk of infection and transmission

Countries	Countries with risk of yellow fever transmission*	Countries requiring yellow fever vaccination for travellers coming from countries with risk of yellow fever transmission*	Countries requiring yellow fever vaccination for travellers from all countries
Botswana		Yes	
Brazil	Yes	Yes	
Brunei Darussalam		Yes	
Burkina Faso	Yes		Yes
Burundi	Yes	Yes	
Cambodia		Yes	
Cameroon	Yes		Yes
Cape Verde		Yes	
Central African Republic	Yes		Yes
Chad	Yes	Yes	
China		Yes	
Christmas Island		Yes	
Colombia	Yes		
Congo	Yes		Yes
Congo, Democratic Republic of	Yes		Yes
Côte d'Ivoire	Yes		Yes
Djibouti		Yes	
Dominica		Yes	
Ecuador	Yes	Yes	
Egypt		Yes	
El Salvador		Yes	

* Either yellow fever has been reported or disease in the past plus presence of vectors and animal reservoirs create a potential risk of infection and transmission

207

Countries	Countries with risk of yellow fever transmission*	Countries requiring yellow fever vaccination for travellers coming from countries with risk of yellow fever transmission*	Countries requiring yellow fever vaccination for travellers from all countries
Equatorial Guinea	Yes	Yes	
Eritrea		Yes	
Ethiopia	Yes	Yes	
Fiji		Yes	
French Guyana	Yes		Yes
French Polynesia		Yes	
Gabon	Yes		Yes
Gambia	Yes	Yes	
Ghana	Yes		Yes
Grenada		Yes	
Guadeloupe		Yes	
Guatemala		Yes	
Guinea	Yes	Yes	
Guinea-Bissau	Yes	Yes	
Guyana	Yes	Yes	
Haiti		Yes	
Honduras		Yes	
India		Yes	
Indonesia		Yes	
Iran		Yes	
Iraq		Yes	
Jamaica		Yes	

*   Either yellow fever has been reported or disease in the past plus presence of vectors and animal reservoirs create a potential risk of infection and transmission

Countries	Countries with risk of yellow fever transmission*	Countries requiring yellow fever vaccination for travellers coming from countries with risk of yellow fever transmission*	Countries requiring yellow fever vaccination for travellers from all countries
Jordan		Yes	
Kazakhstan		Yes	
Kenya	Yes	Yes	
Kiribati		Yes	
Lao People's Democratic Republic		Yes	
Lebanon		Yes	
Lesotho		Yes	
Liberia	Yes	Yes	
Libyan Arab Jamahiriya		Yes	
Madagascar		Yes	
Malawi		Yes	
Malaysia		Yes	
Maldives		Yes	
Mali	Yes	Yes	
Malta		Yes	
Mauritania	Yes	Yes	
Mauritius		Yes	
Montserrat		Yes	
Mozambique		Yes	
Myanmar		Yes	
Namibia		Yes	

* Either yellow fever has been reported or disease in the past plus presence of vectors and animal reservoirs create a potential risk of infection and transmission

Countries	Countries with risk of yellow fever transmission*	Countries requiring yellow fever vaccination for travellers coming from countries with risk of yellow fever transmission*	Countries requiring yellow fever vaccination for travellers from all countries
Nauru		Yes	
Nepal		Yes	
Netherlands Antilles		Yes	
New Caledonia		Yes	
Nicaragua		Yes	
Niger	Yes		Yes
Nigeria	Yes	Yes	
Niue		Yes	
Oman		Yes	
Pakistan		Yes	
Palau		Yes	
Panama	Yes	Yes	
Papua New Guinea		Yes	
Paraguay		Yes	
Peru	Yes		
Philippines		Yes	
Pitcairn Islands		Yes	
Portugal		Yes	
Reunion		Yes	
Rwanda	Yes		Yes
Saint Helena		Yes	
Saint Kitts and Nevis		Yes	

* Either yellow fever has been reported or disease in the past plus presence of vectors and animal reservoirs create a potential risk of infection and transmission

Countries	Countries with risk of yellow fever transmission*	Countries requiring yellow fever vaccination for travellers coming from countries with risk of yellow fever transmission*	Countries requiring yellow fever vaccination for travellers from all countries
Saint Lucia		Yes	
Saint Vincent and the Grenadines	Yes		
Samoa		Yes	
Sao Tome and Principe	Yes		Yes
Saudi Arabia		Yes	
Senegal	Yes	Yes	
Seychelles		Yes	
Sierra Leone	Yes		Yes
Singapore		Yes	
Solomon Islands		Yes	
Somalia	Yes	Yes	
South Africa		Yes	
Sri Lanka		Yes	
Sudan	Yes	Yes	
Suriname	Yes	Yes	
Swaziland		Yes	
Syrian Arab Republic		Yes	
Tanzania, United Republic of	Yes	Yes	
Thailand		Yes	
Timor Leste		Yes	

* Either yellow fever has been reported or disease in the past plus presence of vectors and animal reservoirs create a potential risk of infection and transmission

Countries	Countries with risk of yellow fever transmission*	Countries requiring yellow fever vaccination for travellers coming from countries with risk of yellow fever transmission*	Countries requiring yellow fever vaccination for travellers from all countries
Togo	Yes		Yes
Tonga		Yes	
Trinidad and Tobago	Yes	Yes	
Tunisia		Yes	
Uganda	Yes	Yes	
Uruguay		Yes	
Venezuela	Yes		
Viet Nam		Yes	
Yemen		Yes	
Zimbabwe		Yes	

* Either yellow fever has been reported or disease in the past plus presence of vectors and animal reservoirs create a potential risk of infection and transmission

International Health Regulations

The spread of infectious diseases from one part of the world to another is not a new phenomenon, but in recent decades a number of factors have underscored the fact that infectious disease events in one country may be of potential concern for the entire world. These factors include: increased population movements, whether through tourism or migration or as a result of disasters; growth in international trade in food; biological, social and environmental changes linked with urbanization; deforestation; alterations in climate; and changes in methods of food processing, distribution and consumer habits. Consequently, the need for international cooperation in order to safeguard global health has become increasingly important.

The International Health Regulations (IHR), adopted in 1969, amended in 1973 and 1981[1] and completely revised in 2005[2] provide the legal framework for such international cooperation. The stated purpose of the Regulations is to prevent, protect against, control and provide public health responses to the international spread of disease in ways that are commensurate with and restricted to public health risks, and which avoid unnecessary interference with international traffic and trade.

Their main objectives are to ensure: (1) the appropriate application of routine, preventive measures (e.g. at ports and airports) and the use by all countries of internationally approved documents (e.g. vaccination certificates); and (2) the notification to WHO of all events that may constitute a public health emergency of international concern; and (3) the implementation of any temporary recommendations should the WHO Director-General have determined that such an emergency is occurring. In addition to its new notification and reporting requirements, the IHR (2005) focus on the provision of support for affected states and the avoidance of stigma and unnecessary negative impact on international travel and trade.

---

[1] *International Health Regulations (1969): third annotated edition.* Geneva, World Health Organization, 1983.

[2] *International Health Regulations (2005)*: http://www.who.int/csr/ihr/en/

The IHR (2005) enter into force on 15 June 2007. They take account of the present volume of international traffic and trade and current trends in the epidemiology of infectious diseases, as well as other emerging and re-emerging health risks.

The two specific applications of the IHR (2005) most likely to be encountered by travellers are the yellow fever vaccination requirements imposed by certain countries (see Chapter 6; country list) and the disinsection of aircraft to prevent importation of disease vectors (see Chapter 2).

The vaccination requirements and the disinsection measures are intended to help prevent the international spread of diseases and, in the context of international travel, to do so with the minimum inconvenience to the traveller. This requires international collaboration in the detection and reduction or elimination of the sources of infection.

Ultimately, the risk of an infectious agent becoming established in a country is determined by the quality of the national epidemiological and public health capacities and, in particular, by day-to-day national health and disease surveillance activities and the ability to detect and implement prompt and effective control measures. The requirements for states to establish certain minimum capacities in this regard will, when implemented, provide increased security for visitors as well as for the resident population of the country.

Index of countries and territories

Index by subject